# Medical Robotics - New Achievements

*Edited by Serdar Küçük and Abdullah Erdem Canda*

Published in London, United Kingdom

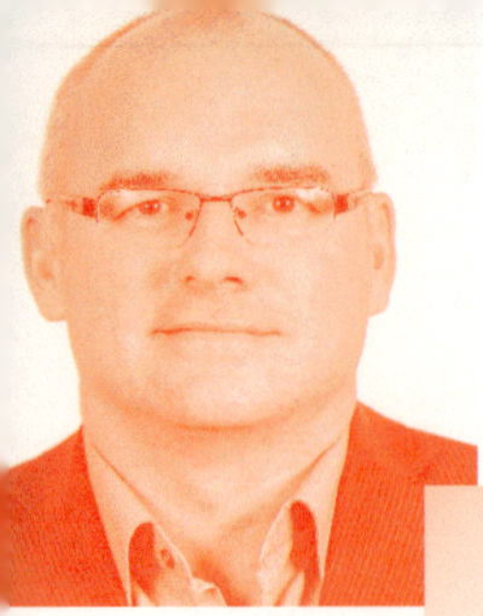
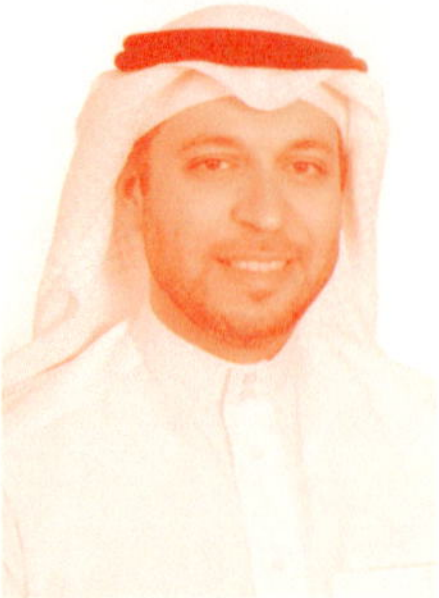
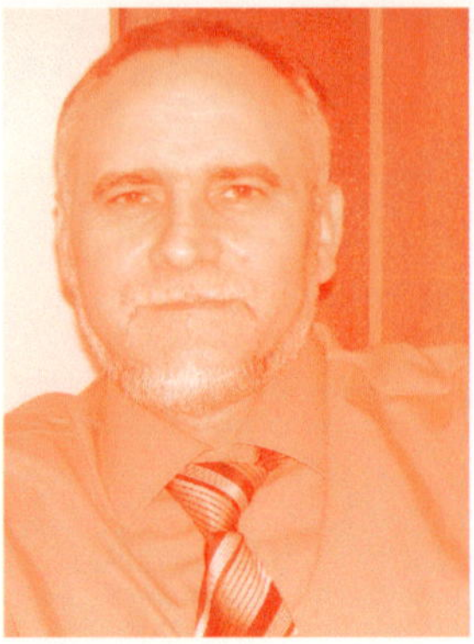
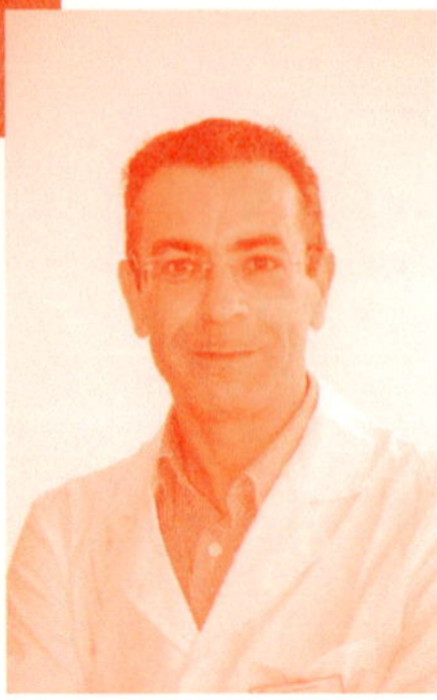
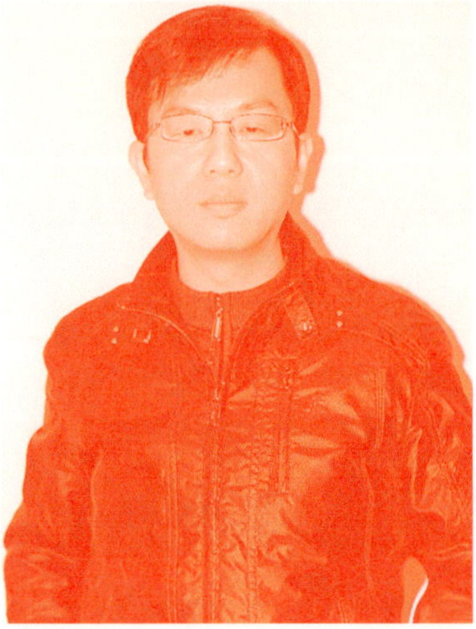
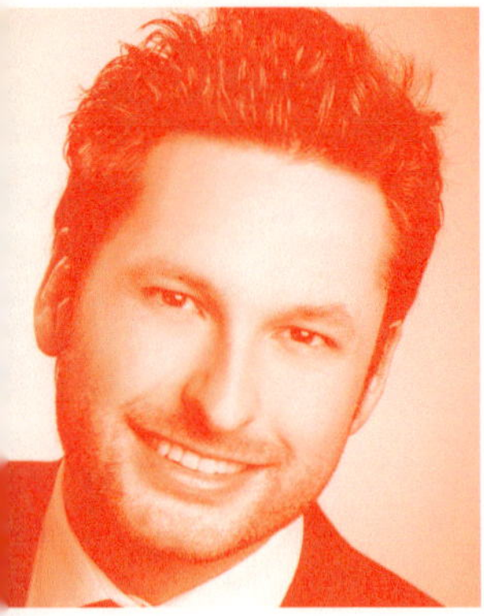
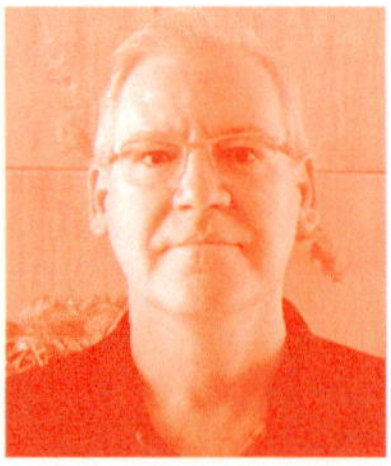

IntechOpen

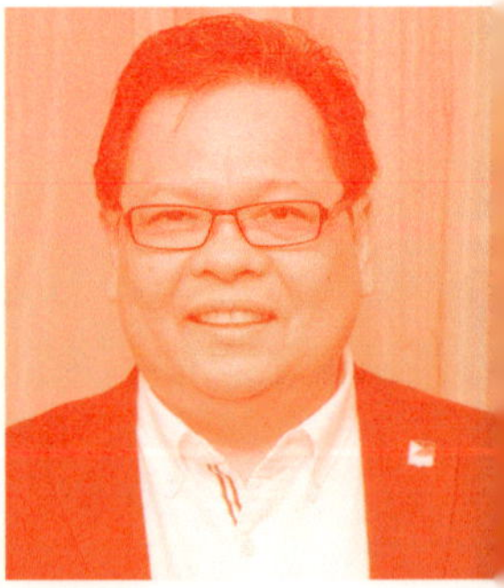
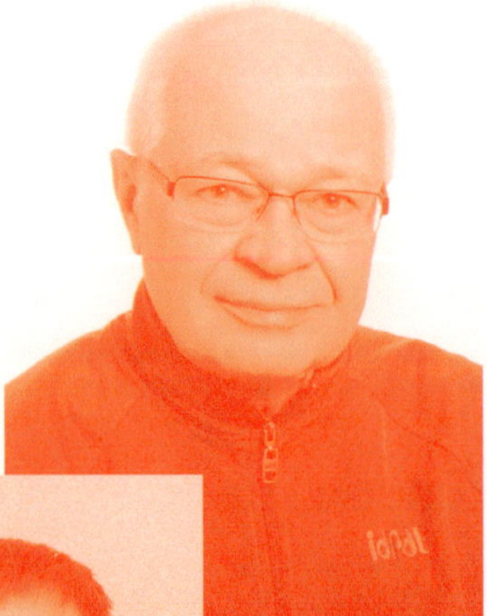
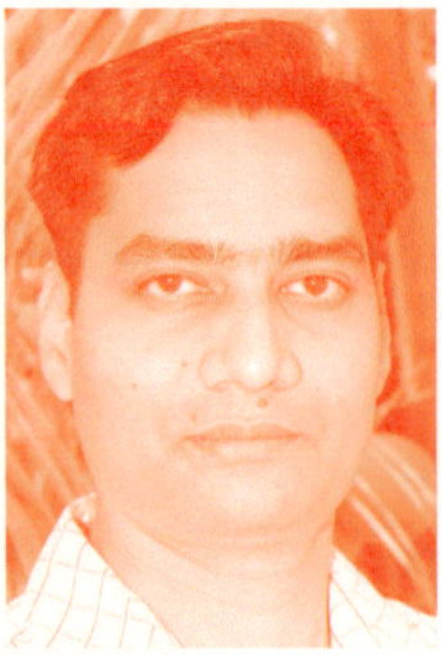
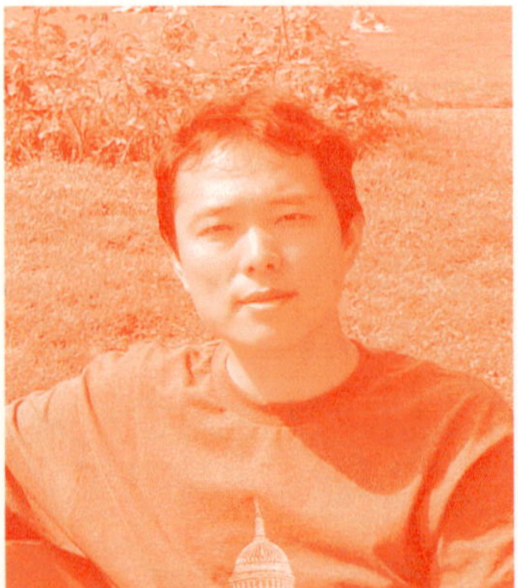
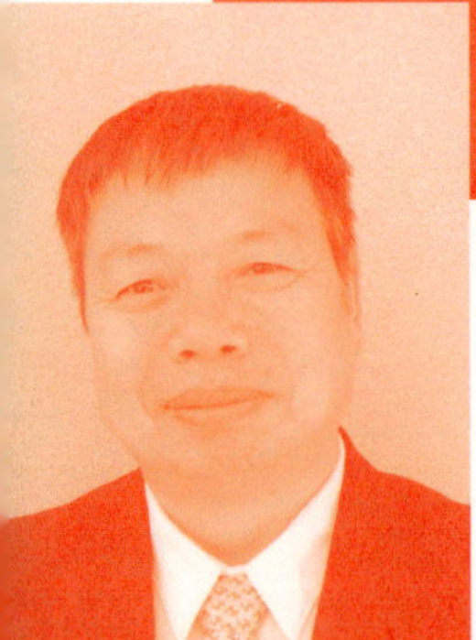
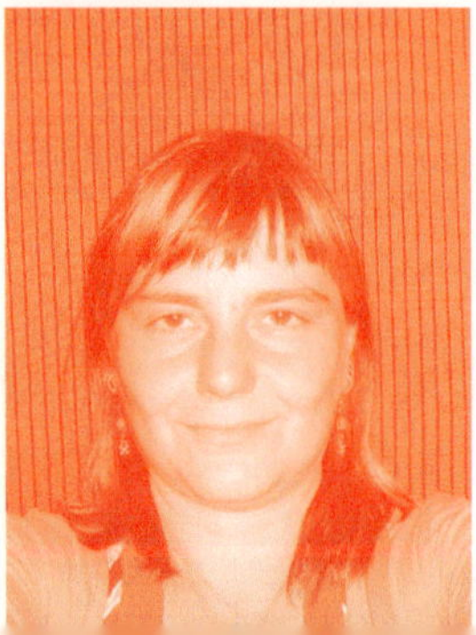

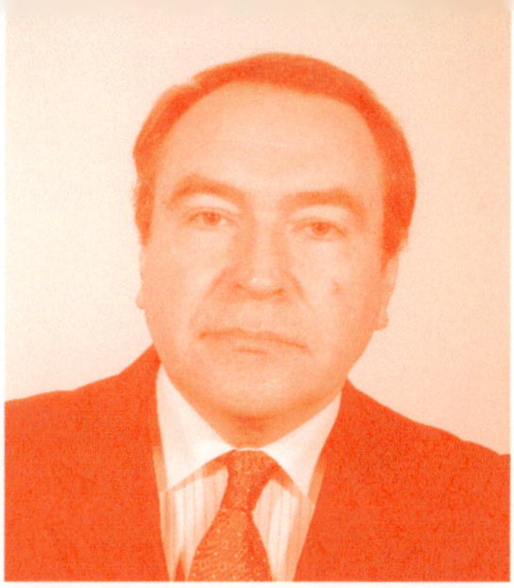
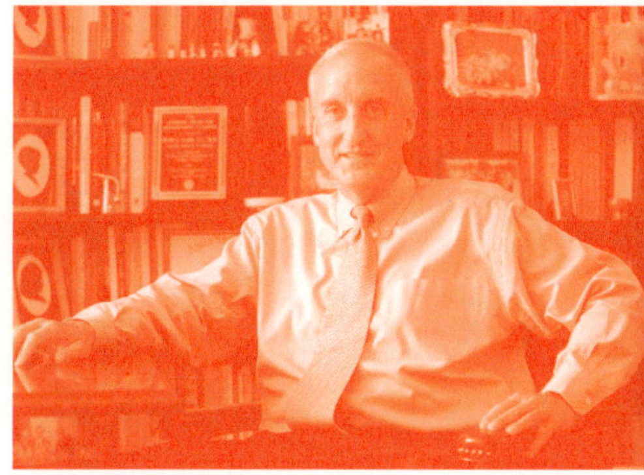
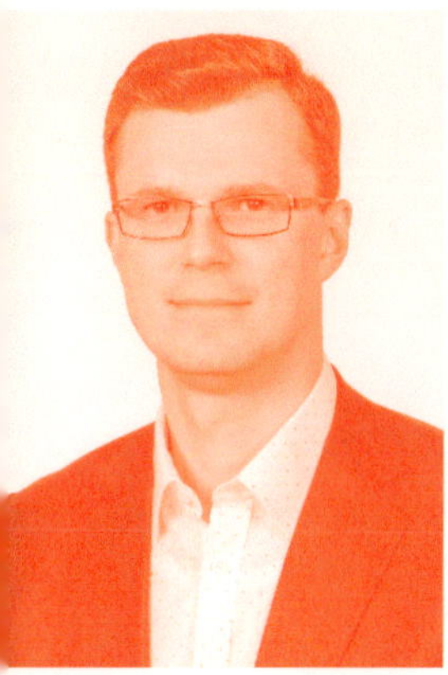
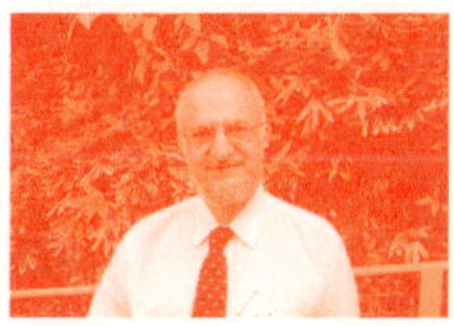
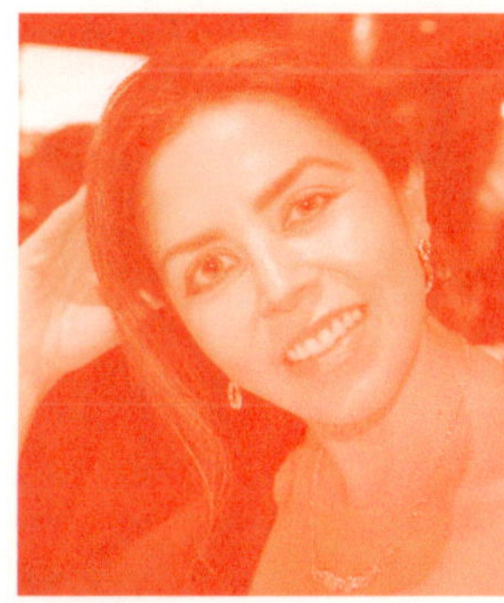

*Supporting open minds since 2005*

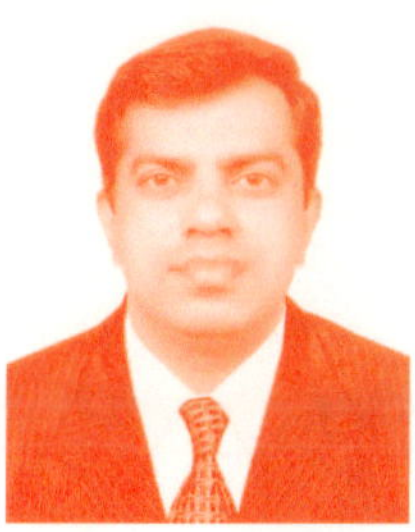
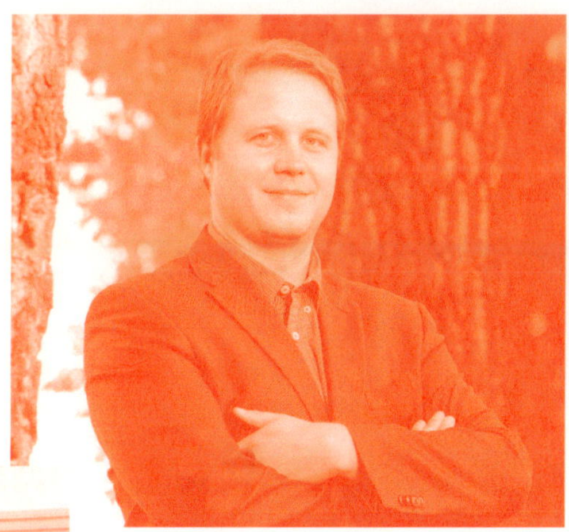
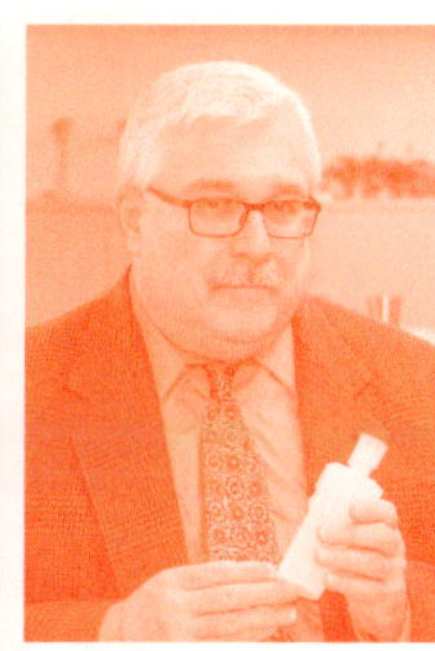
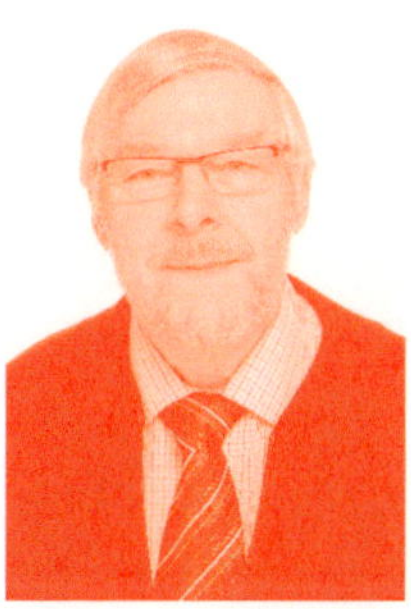
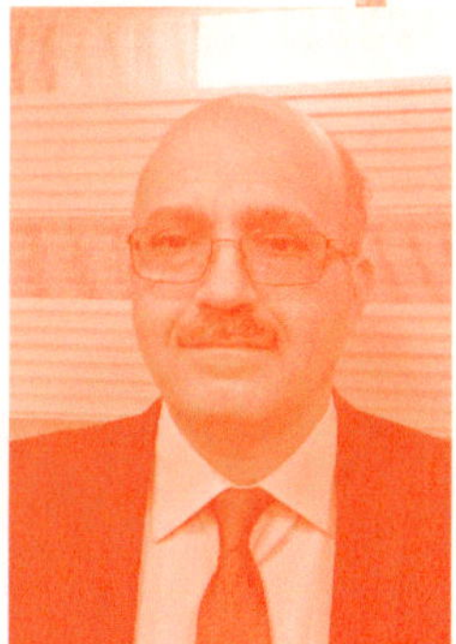
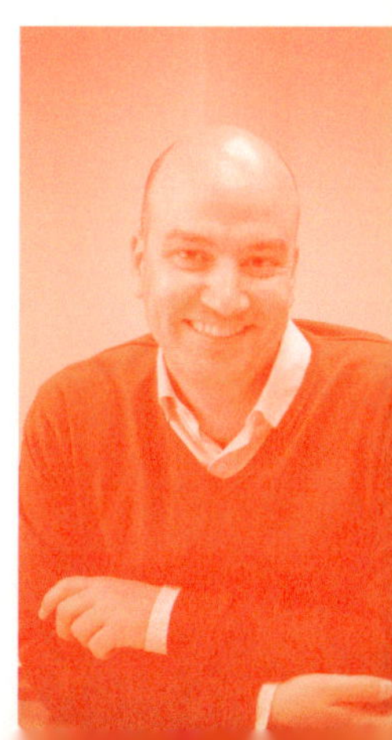
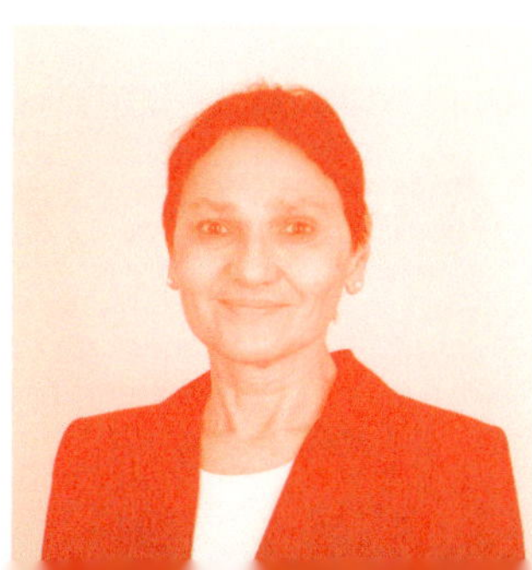

Medical Robotics - New Achievements
http://dx.doi.org/10.5772/intechopen.75257
Edited by Serdar Küçük and Abdullah Erdem Canda

Contributors
Hirofumi Tanabe, Toshimasa Mikawa, Munehiro Ikuta, Akihiko Kondo, Yoshifumi Morita, Alexander Aloy, Simon Hell, Andreas Nowak, Matthaeus Grasl, Serdar Küçük, Kyu-Sung Lee, Kwang Jin Ko, Nicolo'Maria Buffi, Pietro Diana, Paolo Casale, Alberto Saita, Victor Enrique Corona-Montes, Eduardo Gonzalez-Cuenca, Marcos Tobias Machado, Benjamin Van Parys, Karel Decaestecker, Liesbeth Desender, Alberto Breda, Angelo Territo, Ricardo Campi, Giulio Bevilacqua, Mucahit Ege, Levent Aydin, Gabriella Eula, Elisabetta Geda, Giuliano Carlo Geminiani, Silvia Appendino, Terenziano Raparelli, Silvia Sirolli, Guido Belforte, Marina Zettin, Roberta Virgilio, Katiuscia Sacco



First published in London, United Kingdom, 2020 by IntechOpen
IntechOpen is the global imprint of INTECHOPEN LIMITED, registered in England and Wales, registration number: 11086078, 7th floor, 10 Lower Thames Street, London, EC3R 6AF, United Kingdom
Printed in Croatia

British Library Cataloguing-in-Publication Data
A catalogue record for this book is available from the British Library

Additional hard and PDF copies can be obtained from orders@intechopen.com

Medical Robotics - New Achievements
Edited by Serdar Küçük and Abdullah Erdem Canda
p. cm.
Print ISBN 978-1-83968-495-1
Online ISBN 978-1-83968-496-8
eBook (PDF) ISBN 978-1-83968-497-5

For EU product safety concerns:
IN TECH d.o.o., Prolaz Marije Krucifikse Kozulić 3, 51000 Rijeka, Croatia, info@intechopen.com or visit our website at intechopen.com.

# Meet the editors

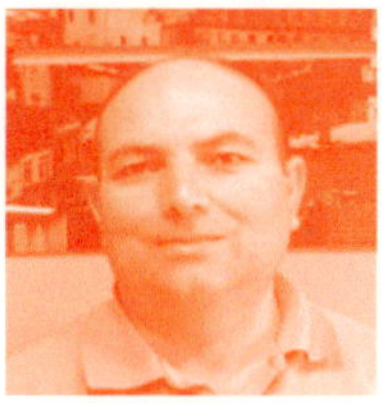

Serdar Küçük obtained BA and MSc degrees from Marmara University (Istanbul, Turkey) in 1995 and 1998, respectively. He obtained his PhD from Kocaeli University (Kocaeli, Turkey) in 2004. He is currently working as a full professor in the Department of Biomedical Engineering at Kocaeli University. He has several scientific publications including international conference papers, journal papers, books, and book chapters. He serves as a reviewer for several well-known robotic journals. He has also edited scientific books. Dr. Kucuk's research interests include optimization, control, kinematics, and dynamics modelling of serial and parallel robotic manipulators. Lately he has also been interested in designing electrically controlled above-knee prosthetics and hand-wrist rehabilitation robots, surgical robots, and biomedical devices.

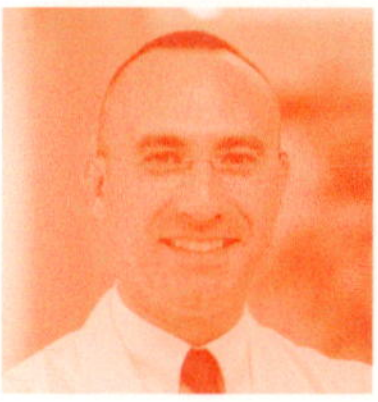

Prof. Canda was born in Izmir, Turkey in 1974. He graduated from Hacettepe University, School of Medicine, Ankara, Turkey, and completed his residency at Dokuz Eylul University, School of Medicine, Department of Urology, Izmir, Turkey. During his residency, Dr. Canda spent two months in the Department of Urology, Catholic University of Leuven, Leuven, Belgium, for uro-oncological training. He had clinical and research fellowships at the University of Sheffield, Department of Biomedical Sciences; the Royal Hallamshire Hospital, Department of Urology; and the Bristol Urological Institute at Southmead Hospital. He also had a three-month fellowship in Laparoscopic Urology at the University of Heidelberg, SLK Kliniken Heilbronn, Department of Urology, Heilbronn, Germany. Between 2008 and 2018, he worked at Ankara Ataturk Training and Research Hospital and Ankara Yildirim Beyazit University in academic positions. Since 2018, he has been working at Koç University, School of Medicine, Istanbul, Turkey. His main interest is robotic urology, and he has been performing robotic urology since 2009. He has personal experience with and exposure to more than 1000 robotic urological surgical cases. He has particular expertise in robotic prostate cancer, kidney cancer, and bladder cancer surgeries. He is an editorial board member of *European Urology*, the Videourology section editor for *Central European Journal of Urology*, editor of *European Medical Journal-Urology*, and editorial board member of *Robotic Surgery Research and Reviews*. He is a board member of the European Association of Urology (EAU) Robotic Urology Section (ERUS) and previously served as a junior-ERUS board member. He is a reviewer for many international, peer-reviewed scientific journals. He has published many international and national papers, particularly on robotic urology. He has received many awards for presentations during congresses on robotic urology.

# Contents

# Preface

Two or three decades ago, robots were considered science fiction. They performed several fantastic tasks only in the movies. Robotic technology has developed very quickly and what was once considered "science fiction" has now become reality. Nowadays robots can execute several kinds of different tasks in factories and are used to manage vital operations in hospitals. Robotic systems have evolved to such a point that they can work together with humans in factories, hospitals, and other organizations. Humans sometimes worry that in the future robots may take their jobs.

Robotic manipulators are used in both industry and medicine. In industry, robots are used for several tasks such as painting, welding, gluing, spraying, and so on. They are used in industry because they present several advantages like reduced manufacturing time, consistent accuracy, and very high product quality. Robots are also used in medicine for several purposes. Surgery and rehabilitation are two major areas in which robots are extensively employed. Surgical robots are preferred since they present better results compared to traditional methods, such as decreased blood loss, less requirement of blood transfusion, decreased rate of complications, smaller incisions, higher accuracy, and lesser recovery time. Although the history of surgical robots is very short compared to the history of surgery, thousands of surgical robots have been installed at hospitals worldwide, and hundreds of thousands of people have been treated by them. The present state of surgical robotics amazes both medical specialists and patients and therefore it is worth it to follow up with new designs and approaches of surgical robots and instruments in the future. Rehabilitation robots are especially used for assisting different types of sensorimotor functions in the arms, hands, and legs. It has been shown that patients are becoming more familiar and comfortable with rehabilitation robots as the technology presents better opportunities and devices every day. Each year several new robotic designs are developed for assisting individuals from children to the elderly. This book critically examines the development and historical evolution of medical robotics with a particular focus on urologic robotic surgery.

I would like to thank all authors who have contributed chapters with their valuable novel ideas and their knowledge on current developments about medical robotics and instruments.


**Serdar Küçük, PhD**
Full Professor,
Kocaeli University,
Technology Faculty,
Department of Biomedical Engineering,
Turkey

**Abdullah Erdem Canda**
Professor,
Koç University,
Turkey

Section 1

# Introduction

Chapter 1

# Introductory Chapter: Medical Robots in Surgery and Rehabilitation

*Serdar Kucuk*

## 1. Introduction

After development of the first advanced robot, they have rapidly become a part of human life. Nowadays robots are smart enough to perform a task in factories, manage an operation in hospitals, and find their way in big shopping centers. The development in automaton and robotic technology are now inevitable. In every passing day, new inventions have been made, and people have come to such a point that they work together with a robot in an organization. Even they are doubtful for a future that a robot may take their jobs. Developments in automation made medical robots enter to several fields of medicine especially surgery and rehabilitation. In the near future, a robot may be a member of hospital staff. Compared to traditional methods, medical robots serve significant advantages to the patients such as better diagnostics, smaller incision, higher accuracy, lesser infection risk, shorter healing time, and longer lifetime.

The development of medical robots can shortly be examined considering three progressive generations, namely, the first-generation robots (like PUMA, Scara, and Delta), second-generation robots (like AESOP), and third-generation robots (like the da Vinci Surgical System). The first-generation robots have not been designed especially for medical purposes. They have been modified for performing medical tasks. The first operation was conducted in 1985 by using PUMA 560 robot manipulator which has a surgical arm mounted on its end effector. A successful neurosurgical biopsy was performed by this manipulator. This operation encourages the robotic experts to design new-generation robots for medicine. On the contrary with the first-generation robots, the second-generation medical robots have especially been designed for medical purposes. AESOP is in the second-generation medical robots. In 1990, AESOP produced by Computer Motion was the first robotic system approved by the Food and Drug Administration (FDA) for medical operations. The third-generation robotic manipulators have been designed and manufactured after the 2000s. These robotic manipulators like the da Vinci Surgical System have been developed especially executing challenging surgical and medical operations. Although the most challenging robots have been developed for surgery operations and people in the world interested mostly in these remarkable robotic systems, robotic rehabilitation devices have also been receiving increasing attention from both medical community and patients. In this chapter, the current status and designs of robotic systems in two major fields (surgery and rehabilitation) are going to be shortly described.

## 2. Medical robots in surgery

It may not be wrong to say that the most challenging robots have been developed for surgery operations since robotic surgery (also called as robotic-assisted surgery) includes many types of dangerous procedures that can be executed with full concentration. Robotic surgery is performed in a tiny incision, and the robot must be continuously under the control of the surgeon. In general, a robotic surgical system possesses arms equipped by camera and surgical instruments and a computer console near the surgical robot or operating table. The surgeon controls each arm of the surgical robotic system by using the computer console that provides surgeon many times magnified 3D view of the operation area. In conventional surgery, surgical operations sometimes take several hours, and the surgeon performs these operations at standing position. This makes the surgeon very tired and loses the surgeon's attention. On the other hand in robotic-assisted surgery, the surgeon sits on a chair and manages other medical staff in his or her chair during the surgical operation. This prevents losing the surgeon's attention to the operation. The other advantages of robotic-assisted surgery compared to the conventional surgical operation can be summarized as follows: smaller incision, lesser pain and blood loss, lesser infection risk, and shorter healing time.

One of the most important surgical robotic systems is without a doubt the da Vinci Surgical System that has been used in millions of operation since its first approval by FDA in 2000. Until now, the da Vinci Surgical System has been used in several different types of operations such as cardiac surgery, colorectal surgery, general surgery, gynecologic surgery, head and neck surgery, thoracic surgery, and urologic surgery [1]. While performing operations with the da Vinci Surgical System, the surgeon sits in front of a console and controls the four interactive robotic arms which are used for holding objects as well as act as scalpels (a little and very sharp-bladed instrument used especially for surgery operations), scissors, and graspers. The surgeon's hand movements are translated into small actions of the instruments mentioned above inside the patient's body. One of the robotic arms holds a camera and a light source which guide the surgeon during the surgery. When the surgeon moves away his head from the console, the activities of da Vinci Surgical System suddenly are stopped. Therefore any severe problem in surgery operation is prevented. da Vinci Surgical System has also some other safety features found in [2].

## 3. Medical robots in rehabilitation

Rehabilitation aims to help patients retain their lost abilities back and return their healthy daily life again. Robotic rehabilitation provides patents to perform some specific exercises to gain abilities back. Rehabilitation robots are especially used for assisting different types of sensorimotor functions like arms, hands, and legs. It has been shown that patients become familiar of rehabilitation robots day by day as the technology offers better opportunities and advanced rehabilitation robotic systems. Robotic rehabilitation can be classified in two major sections, namely, upper extremity rehabilitation and lower extremity rehabilitation. There are several types of robotic systems designed and manufactured for both upper and lower extremity rehabilitation.

### 3.1 Upper extremity robotic rehabilitation devices

The motor functions in upper extremity parts (shoulder, elbow, or writs) can be lost from several types of events such as sports injuries, trauma, occupational injuries [3–5], cerebral palsy in childhood, and stroke in adulthood [6]. This impairment in upper extremity deteriorates the patient's life in many ways such as socially and economically. Therefore it is very important for patients to recover their motor functions and return to their daily life as fast as possible. The number of patients damaged from upper extremity parts is quite high. On the other hand, the number of rehabilitation therapists at the hospitals is very low at present. Therefore it is not possible for rehabilitation therapists to heal all of these patients at current situation. One more difficulty for the patients is that rehabilitation therapies are quite expensive; therefore, it is very difficult to afford. Robotic rehabilitation devices are the potential candidates to recover all of the patient's lost motor functions although they are not extensively commercial at present in the world. It may be said that the manufacturing of more and cheaper robotic rehabilitation devices is a necessity to serve all the patients.

Upper extremity robotic rehabilitation devices have been started to be developed in the beginning of the 1990s [7]. Several upper extremity robotic rehabilitation devices have been designed since the 1990s. Some important points taken into account while designing robotic rehabilitation devices can be summarized as cheap, low mass, compactness, safe operation, easy wearing, portability, and home use [8]. Some recent upper extremity robotic rehabilitation devices can be described as follows: Mit-Manus [9], Reharob [10], Armin [11], Caden-7 [12], Medarm [13], Esa human arm exoskeleton [14], L-exos [15], Armor [16], and Sarcos Master Arm [17]. As can be seen from above studies, several upper extremity robotic rehabilitation devices have been developed as prototypes in general. The number of commercialized robotic rehabilitation devices is still very low compared to the number of patients.

### 3.2 Lower extremity robotic rehabilitation devices

Lower extremity robotic rehabilitation devices can be classified as treadmill gait trainers, footplate-based gait trainers, overground gait trainers, stationary gait and ankle trainers, and active foot orthoses trainers [18]. Diaz et al. [18] summarize the principles of the rehabilitation methods mentioned above in detail.

There are several lower extremity robotic rehabilitation devices that have been built until now. Some of them can be listed as follows: Alex [19], Altraco [20], Arthur [21], LokoHelp [22], Lokomat [23], Lopez [24], ReoAmbulator [25], and String-Man [26]. Although there are several lower extremity robotic rehabilitation devices developed as prototypes or for scientific research purposes, only Lokohelp [22], Lokomat [23], and ReoAmbulator [25] have been commercialized. One of the well-known commercialized lower extremity robotic rehabilitation devices LokoHelp is an electromechanical gait device and trains neurological patients with impaired walking ability [22]. LokoHelp has been tested in several training sessions, and results illustrate that LokoHelp as a robotics rehabilitation system is feasible in severely affected people having brain injury, stroke, and spinal cord injury [22].

The other well-known robot-assisted gait trainer Lokomat composes of a treadmill, a body weight support system, and a robotic gate orthosis. It helps severely impaired neurological patients. The studies illustrates that Lokomat provides effective training and high percentages of recovery potential [23]. The last commercialized lower extremity robotic rehabilitation device is ReoAmbulator that is also a body weight-supported treadmill robotic system [25].

## 4. Conclusion

In this chapter, the designs and current status of medical robots developed for surgery and lower and upper limb rehabilitation have been described. Although the history of both surgical and rehabilitation robotic systems are very short, hundreds of thousands of people have been treated by these robotic systems. The present state of especially surgical robotics amazes both the medical society and the patients. On the other hand, patients become familiar of rehabilitation robots as the technology presents better opportunities like cheaper and more useful designs. Every year new robotic designs for both surgical and rehabilitation purposes are developed for individuals from children to elderly people. As a last word, it is worthy to follow up the new designs and approaches on surgical and rehabilitation robots in the future.

## Author details

Serdar Kucuk
Kocaeli University, Turkey

*Address all correspondence to: skucuk@kocaeli.edu.tr

## References

[1] Dwivedi J, Mahgoub I. Robotic surgery - A review on recent advances in surgical robotic systems, Florida Conference on Recent Advances in Robotics, 2012. Boca Raton, Florida, May 10-11, 2012

[2] Freschi C, Ferrari V, Melfi F, Ferrari M, Mosca F, Cuschieri A. Technical review of the da Vinci surgical telemanipulator. The International Journal of Medical Robotics and Computer Assisted Surgery. Dec 2013;**9**(4):396-406

[3] Reid DC. Sports Injury Assessment and Rehabilitation. New York, NY: Churchill Livingstone; 1992

[4] Mehta JA, Bain GI. Elbow dislocations in adults and children. Clinics in Sports Medicine. 2004;**23**:609-627

[5] Dodson CC, Cordasco FA. Anterior glenohumeral joint dislocations. The Orthopedic Clinics of North America. 2008;**39**:507-518

[6] Mayetin U, Kucuk S, Sade SI. A comparative analysis of hand-wrist rehabilitation devices. In: 7th International Conference on Advance Technologies, April 28–May 1, Antalya, Turkey. 2018

[7] Kommu SS. Rehabilitation Robotics. Vienna, Austria: Itech Education and Publishing; 2007

[8] Islam R, Spiewak C, Rahman HM, Fareh R. A brief review on robotic exoskeletons for upper extremity rehabilitation to find the gap between research porotype and commercial type. Advances in Robotics and Automation. 2017;**6**:3

[9] Krebs HI, Hogan N, Volpe BT, Aisen ML, Edelstein L, Diels C. Overview of clinical trials with MIT-MANUS: A robot-aided neuro- rehabilitation facility. Technology and Health Care. 1999;**7**(6):419-423

[10] Fazekas G, Horvath M, Troznai T, Toth A. Robot-mediated upper limb physiotherapy for patients with spastic hemiparesis: A preliminary study. Journal of Rehabilitation Medicine. 2007;**39**(7):580-582

[11] Nef T, Riener R. ARMin—Design of a novel arm rehabilitation robot. In: Proceedings of the 2005 IEEE 9th International Conference on Rehabilitation Robotics, Chicago, IL, USA. 2005. pp. 57-60

[12] Perry JC. Design and development of a 7 degree-of-freedom powered exoskeleton for the upper limb [dissertation]. University of Washington; 2006

[13] Ball SJ, Brown IE, Scott SH. MEDARM: A rehabilitation robot with 5DOF at the shoulder complex. In: IEEE/ASME International Conference on Advanced Intelligent Mechatronics. 2007

[14] Schiele A, Visentin G. The ESA human arm exoskeleton for space robotics telepresence. In: Conference: International Symposium on Artificial Intelligence, Robotics and Automation in Space (iSAIRAS); Nara, Japan. Vol. 7. 2003

[15] Frisoli A, Bergamasco M, Carboncini C, Carboncini C, Rossi B. Robotic assisted rehabilitation in virtual reality with the L-EXOS. Studies in Health Technology and Informatics. 2009;**145**:40-54

[16] Mayr A, Kofler M, Saltuari L. ARMOR: An electromechanical robot for upper limb training following stroke. A prospective randomised controlled pilot study. Handchirurgie, Mikrochirurgie, Plastische Chirurgie. 2008;**40**(1):66-73

[17] Michael Mistry, Peyman Mohajerian, Stefan Schaal, An exoskeleton robot for human arm movement study, 2005 IEEE/RSJ International Conference on Intelligent Robots and Systems (IROS 2005). 2005

[18] Diaz I, Gil JJ, Sanchez E. Lower-limb robotic rehabilitation: Literature review and challenges. Journal of Robotics. 2011;**2011**:1-11

[19] Banala SK, Agrawal SK, Scholz JP. Active leg exoskeleton (ALEX) for gait rehabilitation of motor-impaired patients. In: Proceedings of the 10th IEEE International Conference on Rehabilitation Robotics, (ICORR '07). Noordwijk, The Netherlands; 2007. pp. 401-407

[20] Beyl P, van Damme M, van Ham R, Versluys R, Vanderborght B, Lefeber D. An exoskeleton for gait rehabilitation: Prototype design and control principle. In: Proceedings of the IEEE International Conference on Robotics and Automation, (ICRA '08). Pasadena, CA, USA; 2008. pp. 2037-2042

[21] Reinkensmeyer D, Wynne J, Harkema S. A robotic tool for studying locomotor adaptation and rehabilitation. In: Proceedings of the 2nd Joint Meeting of the IEEE Engineering in Medicine and Biology Society and the Biomedical Engineering Society. Vol. 3. 2002. pp. 2013-2353

[22] Freivogel S, Mehrholz J, Husak-Sotomayor T, Schmalohr D. Gait training with the newly developed "LokoHelp"-system is feasible for non-ambulatory patients after stroke, spinal cord and brain injury. A feasibility study. Brain Injury. 2008;**22**(7-8):625-632

[23] Colombo G, Joerg M, Schreier R, Dietz V. Treadmill training of paraplegic patients using a robotic orthosis. Journal of Rehabilitation Research and Development. 2000;**37**(6):693-700

[24] Veneman JF, Kruidhof R, Hekman EEG, Ekkelenkamp R, Van Asseldonk EHF, Van Der Kooij H. Design and evaluation of the Lopes exoskeleton robot for interactive gait rehabilitation. IEEE Transactions on Neural Systems and Rehabilitation Engineering. 2007;**15**(3):379-386

[25] West GR. Powered gait orthosis and method of utilizing same. 2004. Patent Number 6 689 075

[26] Surdilovic D, Bernhardt R. STRING-MAN: A new wire robot for gait rehabilitation. In: Proceedings of the IEEE International Conference on Robotics and Automation. Vol. 2. 2004. pp. 2031-2036

Section 2

# Medical Devices

Chapter 2

# CFD Analysis of Flow Characteristics in a Jet Laryngoscope and the Different Application Forms of Superimposed Jet Ventilation

*Alexander Aloy, Simon Hell, Andreas Nowak and Matthaeus Grasl*

## Abstract

The superimposed high-frequency jet ventilation is a jet ventilation technique that allows the surgeon to operate in a system open to the outside endoscopic surgery in the area of the vocal cord level. Although the clinical application is uncomplicated, the possible mechanisms of the gas flow in the jet laryngoscope are largely unknown. In the performed calculations for this work, the CFD software package Fluent is used with the preprocessor GAMBIT. After creating the geometry and networking of the jet laryngoscope in the preprocessor GAMBIT, the boundary conditions and input parameters in the solver are defined. This is followed by iterative calculation using Fluent and the tabulation of results. Ventilation is provided by an electronic respirator specially developed for the endoscope. There is a bidirectional gas flow in the jet laryngoscope. The free jet characteristics of the jet beam can be confirmed. Entrainment depends on pressure and on the gas velocity. The arrangement of the nozzles enables jet ventilation in stenosis. CFD analysis enables the representation of a continuous progress of the pressure as well as the representation of the continuous profile of the velocity in the investigated endoscope. Additionally the practical application for intensive care ventilation is shown.

**Keywords:** jet ventilation, superimposed high-frequency jet ventilation (SHFJV), computational fluid dynamics (CFD), laryngeal stenosis, jet respirator, combined high-frequency jet ventilation, flow behavior

## 1. Introduction

Jet ventilation in medicine means the administration of small to the smallest gas volumes (1–2 ml/kilogram per body weight) with a high frequency from a nozzle or special adaptors to ventilate a patient. This ventilation is used in surgical surgery as well as in intensive care medicine. In contrast to the dynamics of a sustained flight jet beam, the jet stream in medical application is only supposed to expand the lung during the inspiratory phase. Thereafter, the expiration should be passively carried out by sifting the air supply. But in the expiratory phase, the air should not be completely exhaled. A positive end-expiratory pressure (PEEP) should prevent a collapse of alveoli. In case of surgery on the larynx as well as in the trachea, both the surgeon and the anesthetist interfere in the same working area. An often used endotracheal tube ensures the mechanical ventilation and, however, represents a massive disability for the surgeon. One possibility is the use of thin endotracheal tubes to provide the surgeon more space for his operational activity. Alternatively, however, techniques were developed in which the gas flows without endotracheal tube through the surgical area directly into the trachea. One possibility is the use of an endoscope in which nozzles for jet ventilation are integrated. The gas emerging from the nozzles flows through the endoscope and through the vocal cord plane into the trachea.

Computational fluid dynamics (CFD), a viable method for analyzing flow behavior, is well established for the investigation [1] of fluid mechanics. In recent years this method has been applied in the medical field to better understanding the behavior of gas currents in the human lung [2, 3]. Furthermore, technical issues related to mechanical ventilation can be solved by CFD. High-frequency ventilation (high-frequency jet ventilation, jet ventilation) is a ventilation technique that is characterized by the application of a small tidal volume through a variable nozzle, usually at high frequency [4]. Jet ventilation enables the transport and administration of small volumes of compressed gas at high pressures through a thin catheter or small metal tubes whose ends have the characteristics of a nozzle. However, the use of tubes or catheters involves the risk of dislocation or kinking, with the subsequent obstruction of the gas flow [5–7].

Superimposed high-frequency jet ventilation (SHFJV) is a simultaneous, combined application of low- and high-frequency jet ventilations [8]. Jet ventilation is characterized by the appearance of some physical effects whose characteristics make them feasible for mechanical ventilation in endoscopic surgery. One of these effects is the free jet character of the gas flow. The respiratory gas is to be transported in an outward open system from the jets through the vocal cord level in the lung. After the exit of the gas from the nozzle, it moves at the SHFJV over a short distance as a free jet in the direction of the vocal cord level. When the gas leaves the nozzle, the energy of the gas is sufficient to produce a forward pressure thrust. The gas then flows with a reduced controllable pressure needed for mechanical ventilation through the endoscope and glottis into the lungs. Another characteristic of this free jet is an entrainment [9] of the surrounding air. Thus, the enriched oxygen gas coming out of the jet is reduced in its concentration. These physical effects are applicable to jet ventilation and in particular for the superimposed high-frequency jet ventilation. Although this technique was initially developed for operations on the vocal cords in adults, the spectrum of this technology has expanded. Thus, this technique is particularly suitable for children, because of the limited space and the difficult working conditions for the surgeon. Furthermore, the operating range has been extended to the subglottic space and tracheal space. The anatomical relationships are not changed. Another crucial aspect is the use of jet ventilation in high-grade stenosis [10, 11]. The localization of these pathological changes which lead to a reduction in cross section for the gas flow can be localized above, directly in the vocal cord or even below. From a medical-technical point of view, it is necessary to administer the gas jet with a higher pressure in order to maintain a sufficient tidal volume behind the stenosis in the lung. At the same time, however, it must be ensured that the applied gas volume behind the stenosis does not lead to hyperinflation of the lungs. Hyperinflation of the lungs can cause barotrauma due to a blockage of the gas outflow. The question that arises is can the pressure behind the stenosis be higher than the pressure before the stenosis, with this ventilation technique? Current clinical results show that in no case a barotrauma occurred even in cases of severe stenosis [12]. However, publicized data on the validation of the general gas behavior and flow patterns within the jet laryngoscopes is still absent in the literature. The aim of this study was to analyze fluid dynamic processes within the jet laryngoscope by a flow simulation. The behavior of the combined low- and high-frequency jets should be investigated in the endoscope. The entrainment of the gas caused by the two jets with the characteristics of free flow is to be analyzed in its behavior. Subsequently, the behavior of the distribution of the flow and the pressure in a stenosis is to be examined. The potential risk for barotrauma using supraglottic jet ventilation in the presence of a stenosis is to be investigated.

## 1.1 Material and methods

### *1.1.1 Jet laryngoscope*

The jet laryngoscope (comp. Carl Reiner, Vienna, Austria) contains two metal jets welded to the side of the endoscope. The jets are directed downward and end at the inside wall of the laryngoscope with an opening into the lumen. The alignment of each jet stream is based on an imaginary center of the distal end of the laryngoscope, implying that this stream is continued along a median line into the trachea. The openings of the jet nozzles are positioned in the upper third of the endoscope and not at the top of the endoscope. An additional line is affixed to the right side of the laryngoscope. This line ends at the tip of the laryngoscope and solely served to pressure monitoring. Two jet streams with different frequencies were applied simultaneously. The continuous high-frequency jet stream is applied during expiration period and superimposed during the inspiratory phase of the low-frequency jet ventilation. The low-frequency jet stream resulted in phased airway pressure changes analogous to conventional ventilation with 12–20 bpm and provided the upper (higher) pressure level. The high-frequency jet stream has a frequency of 100–1500 cycles/min and is creating the lower pressure level corresponding to a positive end-expiratory pressure (PEEP). The released gas has a pressure of 1–1.5 bar, which declines hundredfold upon reaching the vocal cords resulting in a pressure of 10–15 mbar at the distal endoscope opening. The two jet streams are administered by an electronic respirator (**Figure 1**).

### *1.1.2 Geometry of the model*

For creation of a geometry model, GAMBIT software was used. To reduce computing time, minor simplifications to the model had to be made. The entry and exit diameters of the laryngoscope were approximated to an elliptical form (entry, a = 13 mm and b = 8 mm; exit, a = 7 mm and b = 4 mm; a and b are the semiaxes of the ellipses). The nozzles were depicted as section planes in Fluent to ensure accurate depiction of peripheral airflow conditions. The total length of the laryngoscope was 165 mm, and the angle of oxygen entry was 28°, while the distance between nozzle and gas release diameter was 48 mm for low-frequency and 68 mm for high-frequency ventilation. The inner nozzle diameter was 1.7 mm.

### *1.1.3 The network model*

Connection simulation (**Figure 2**) was also done by GAMBIT software in the following manner: Firstly, the segments immediately before and after the

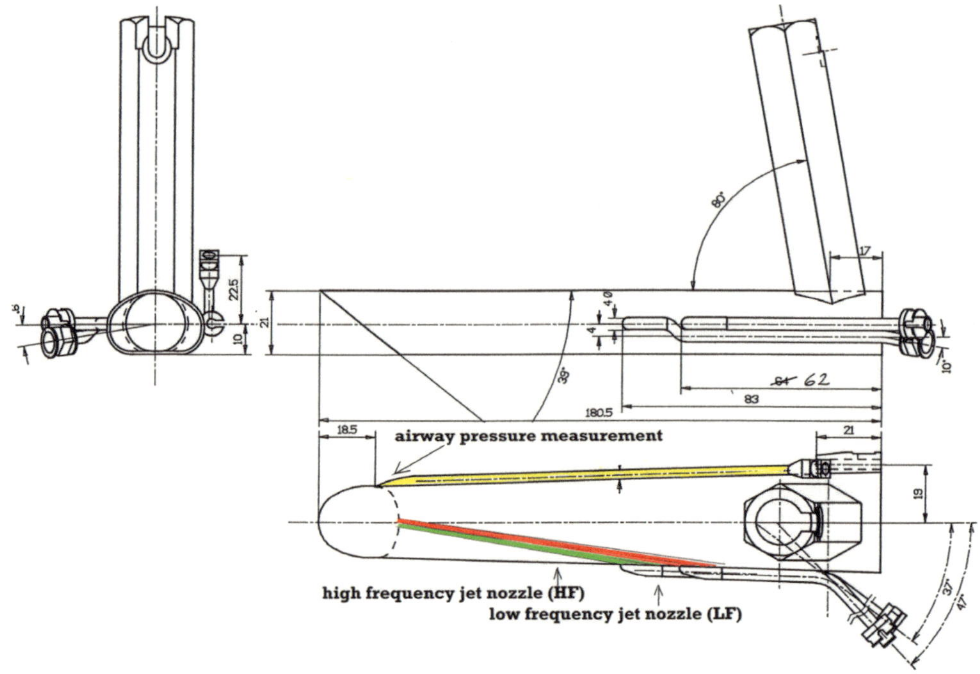


**Figure 1.**
*Schematic description of the jet laryngoscope: Localizations of the jets and airway pressure measurement (yellow).*

laryngoscope entrance and exit diameter were configured according to the Cooper regimen. The front surfaces were connected to the elements of Hex/Hedge type. This implies that hexahedral (six-sided) elements were primarily used, unless wedge elements were required. For the middle segment, the Cooper regimen could not be used, because of the presence of the nozzles. The elements were connected according to the Pave system, which is not compatible with the Cooper regimen. This area around the nozzles was analyzed with higher resolution, because of the essential character of this area for the results of our study. An edge plane was applied to the wall of the laryngoscope.

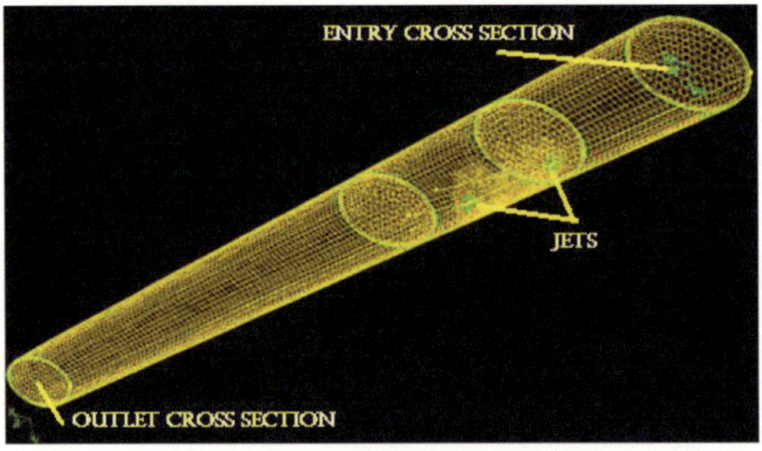


**Figure 2.**
*Networked laryngoscope and 3D geometry.*

The properties and quality of the resulting network are:

- 64.591 nodes, 104.056 volume elements.
- The aspect ratio was limited to a value of <5, except in the outer segments where a ratio of 10 was deemed acceptable (The aspect ratio is only greater than 3.6 in the outer segments.).
- The average skewness factor was limited to 0.33, and the maximum to 0.95 (0.17 and 0.94, respectively).
- The maximal squish index value was 0.99 (0.84).

*1.1.3.1 Fluent*

Fluent is a software solution utilizing the finite volume method to solve the problem at hand. Before the iterative solution process can be undertaken, certain settings with significant relevance need to be defined.

*1.1.3.2 Settings*

*1.1.3.2.1 Solver*

The pressure-based solver was selected.

*1.1.3.2.2 Turbulence model*

Because of the relatively high Reynolds values (44,000 and 28,000) of the laryngoscope entrance and exit zones, the airflow in the laryngoscope is turbulent. For numerical calculation the realizable k-E value was chosen, because the standard κ-ε model was not suited because of its weakness in calculation of sudden acceleration. Finally, the realizable κ-ε model was chosen

*1.1.3.2.3 Species*

Air and pure oxygen were defined as present substance in the presented model to determine the specific oxygen density at the exit diameter. The model allowed for the normal oxygen concentration of pure air (21%), because the Fluent software does not incorporate this correction factor automatically.

*1.1.3.2.4 Boundary conditions*

- Entrance diameter

Pressure inlet with surrounding pressure.

The utilized value is an approximation, due to the fact that the pressure upon entry is not constant, but depends on the pressure of both end stream nozzles. The higher the entrance velocity of the applied gas is, the higher the negative pressure of the entrance diameter becomes.

- Exit diameter

Pressure outlet with an assumed pulmonary pressure of 30/15 mbar

- Jets (nozzles)

Pressure inlet with 0.8 bar pressure at the low-frequency nozzle and 1.3 bar at the high-frequency aperture

- Wall

*1.1.3.2.5 Solution controls*

The settings of iteration, under-relaxation factors, and residuals were adapted to the stage of computation.

*1.1.3.2.6 Steady flow*

The pressures at both jets were assumed to be constant. The following conditions (**Table 1**) were analyzed.

*1.1.3.2.7 Unsteady flow*

The instationary current at the low-frequency nozzle is not constant, but varies between 0 and 1.3 bar, alternating every 2.5 sec. To accommodate this fact, a user-defined function (UDF) was programmed and added to the simulation. The pressure at the high-frequency nozzle was assumed to be constant.

To ensure accurate results for each time interval, each time interval should be short enough. Utilizing the Courant–Friedrichs–Lewy (CFL) value, every time step can be predicted sufficiently. The implied solver should be approximately 10.

$$\Delta t < CFLmin * \frac{\Delta x}{U}$$

$\Delta x$, element length; U, velocity.

Because the net is smallest and the velocity is highest as the nozzle exits, the time interval was estimated according to this data. This computes to $\Delta t$ of 5e–6 s ($\Delta x$ = 0.17 mm, U = 350 m/s), which in turn implies 20.000 intervals per second.

## 2.1 Results

Cases with stationary pressure with different pressure conditions and the effect of a stenosis were simulated. Simultaneous high- and low-frequency jet ventilation (Case A) is applied at an intrapulmonary pressure of 30 mbar. In this case, maximal velocities of 295 m/s could be measured at the low-frequency nozzle. The velocity

| | Pressure (low-frequency jet) [bar] | Pressure (high-frequency jet) [bar] |
|---|---|---|
| Case A | 1.3 | 0.8 |
| Case B | 0 | 0.8 |
| Case C | 1.3 | 0 |

**Table 1.**
*The pressure at both jets was assumed to be constant. The following conditions were analyzed. Case A was defined as the gas current during inspiration and expiration.*

drops rapidly to a value of 43.2 m/s at the laryngoscope exit (**Figure 3**). The vector field (**Figure 4**) of the measured velocities of the high and low frequencies of gas current depicts the gas flow toward the lungs, and the simultaneous exit flows out of the lung contralaterally, allowing for an additional recirculation component on the opposite side of the nozzles. A negative pressure (**Figure 5**) is created due to the free jet characteristic of gas flow directly after having left the nozzle. These results in surround room air are sucked from the open end to the atmosphere.

## 2.2 Change in pulmonary pressure

Further simulation of the flow characteristics inside the jet laryngoscope, assuming a lower pressure in the lung (15 mbar). At first glance it is obvious the velocities along the z-axis rise (**Table 2**) when the opposite force in the lung is lower. The combined application of high- and low-frequency jet ventilation at

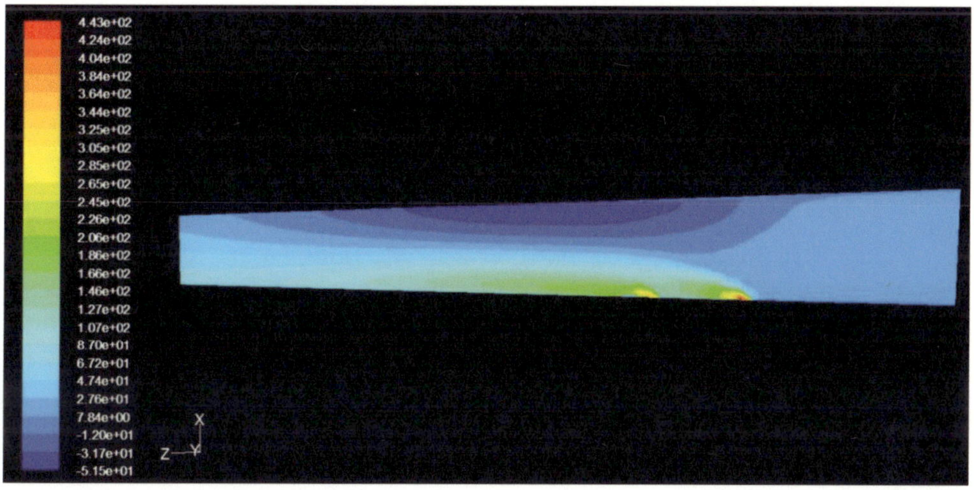


**Figure 3.**
*z-component of velocity distribution (m/s). The influx of the gas takes place starting from the nozzle to the left. On the opposite side is the outflow of the gas.*

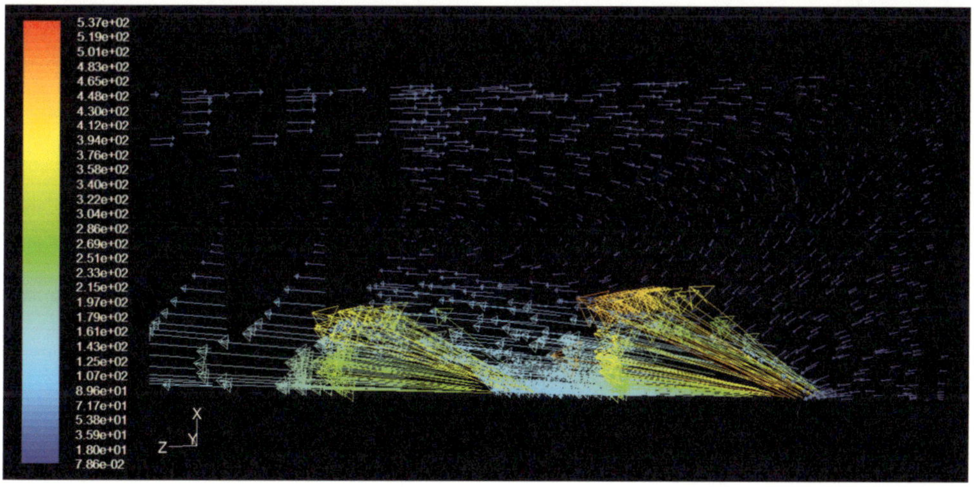


**Figure 4.**
*Vector field of the velocity in the region of the two nozzle (m/s).*

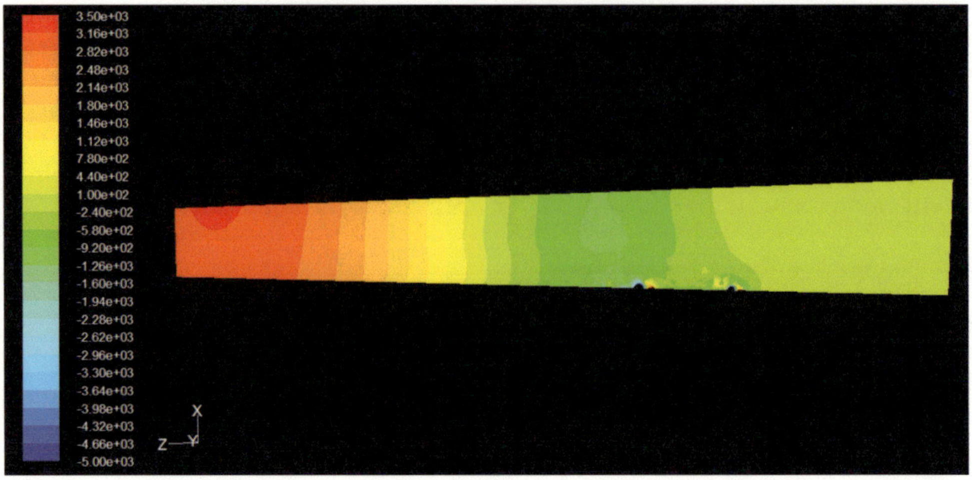


**Figure 5.**
*Pressure distribution (the areas around the nozzles have been excluded due to the strong negative or high positive pressure of the color scale, to ensure that the pressure differences in the remaining region are more visible, pressure in Pa).*

unchanged high "driving pressure" as in Case A shows that, with low pulmonary pressure (15 mbar), the velocities in the entrance and exit zones are markedly higher. Case C of single low-frequency jet ventilation exhibits a higher velocity as the single high-frequency jet (Case B) ventilation. However, the increased gas velocity results in a raised entrainment of air, reducing the oxygen concentration in the exit zone. **Table 3** shows that the mass transport is directly proportional to the velocities. **Figure 6** shows (Case A) the development of the gas flow with a lower intrapulmonary pressure. But here, too, there is a bidirectional gas flow.

## 3. Stenosis

This simulation attempted to imitate laryngeal pathology with stenosis by reducing the cross section at the tip of the laryngoscope. In this study, a short yet circular stenosis was examined (**Figure 7**) similar to a clinical situation. The half-axes of the cross section were reduced from 7 to 4.5 mm and from 4 to 2.5 mm, which meant a reduction of 60% in diameter. For further simulation the system was extended after the stenosis by a piece of pipe. The remaining conditions are identical to Case A (combined high- and low-frequency jet ventilation). The intrapulmonary pressure

| | **v Exit** | **v Exit** | **v Entrance** | **v Entrance** | **$O_2$ Exit** | **$O_2$ Exit** |
|---|---|---|---|---|---|---|
| | **[m/s]** | **[m/s]** | **[m/s]** | **[m/s]** | **[%]** | **[%]** |
| | **15 mbar** | **30 mbar** | **15 mbar** | **30 mbar** | **15 mbar** | **30 mbar** |
| Case A | 58.38 | 43.51 | Dez.89 | | 48 | 53 |
| Case B | 23.27 | −27.09 | Apr.85 | −10.03 | 42 | 22 |
| Case C | 38.99 | 15.55 | Aug.75 | Jän.90 | 50 | 57 |

**Table 2.**
*Comparison of two different lung pressures (15 vs. 30 mbar). Behavior of flow velocities (m/s) and the oxygen content (%) at the entrance and exit of the jet laryngoscope at three different ventilation modes (Cases A, B, and C).*

| | Mass transport in the exit [kg/s] 15 mbar | Mass transport in the exit [kg/s] 30 mbar |
|---|---|---|
| Case A | −0.006892061 | −0.0050869673 |
| Case B | −0.002731038 | 0.003058461 |
| Case C | −0.004529244 | −0.001836674 |

**Table 3.**
*Mass transport at the outlet cross section.*

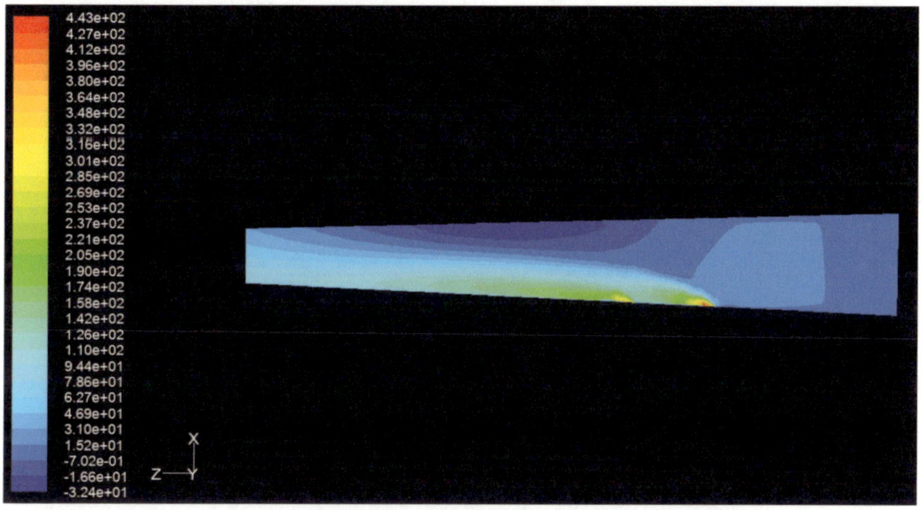


**Figure 6.**
*Velocity distribution for case A at 15 mbar pressure lung (m/s).*

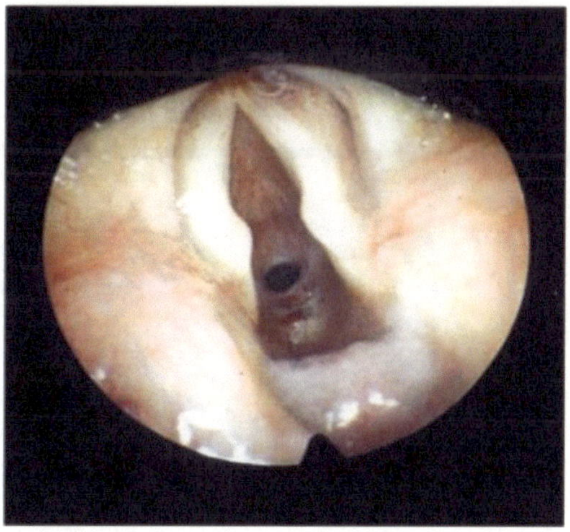

**Figure 7.**
*Clinical situation of a circular stenosis just below the vocal cord level.*

was set at 15 mm. The reduction of ventilation diameter has the following implications: Proximal to stenosis the pressure rises (45 mbar), resulting in a reduction in velocity (approx. 20 m/s) before increasing once again (**Figure 8**) in the region of the stenosis and immediately post-stenotically (70 m/s) until a stable velocity of

25 m/s is reached. Simultaneously, there is a bidirectional gas flow in the laryngoscope again.

(**Figure 9**) shows the pressure distribution at the stenosis. The pre-stenotic pressure corresponds to a dynamic pressure. It is important to note that despite the pre-stenotic pressure being relatively high, there is an obligatory drop in post-stenotic pressure (**Figure 10**). This results in an increase of lateral backflow and in consequence reduced entrainment. (**Figure 11**) shows the vector field of the velocity in the area of stenosis. Localized recirculation can be seen. There is a backflow both before and after the stenosis.

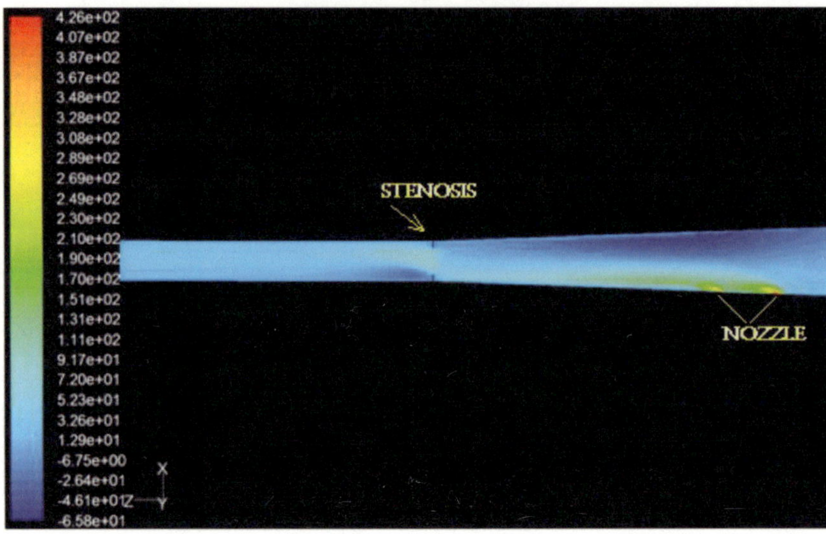


**Figure 8.**
*Velocity distribution in occurring stenosis at a pulmonary pressure from 15 mbar. At the side of the nozzle is a high gas velocity. Simultaneously a gas discharge is on the opposite side (m/sec).*

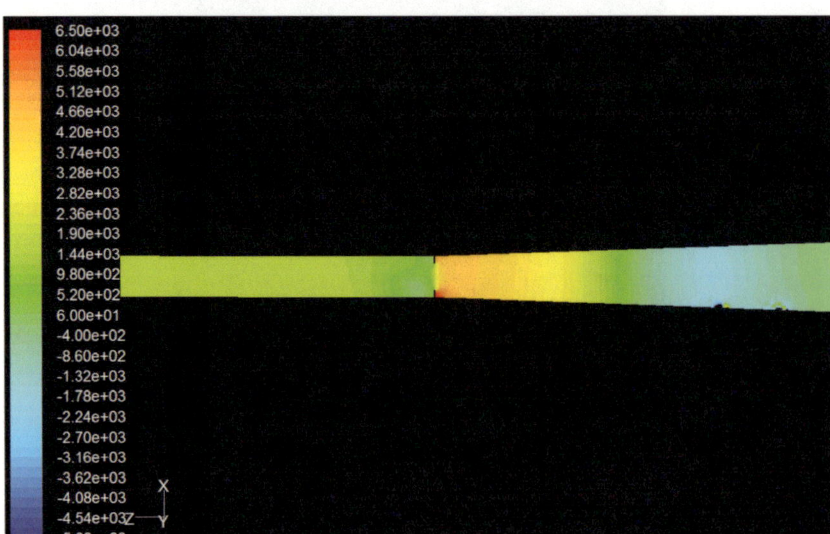


**Figure 9.**
*The pressure increases continuously in front of the stenosis, but he is lower in the area of the stenosis and after the stenosis (Pa).*

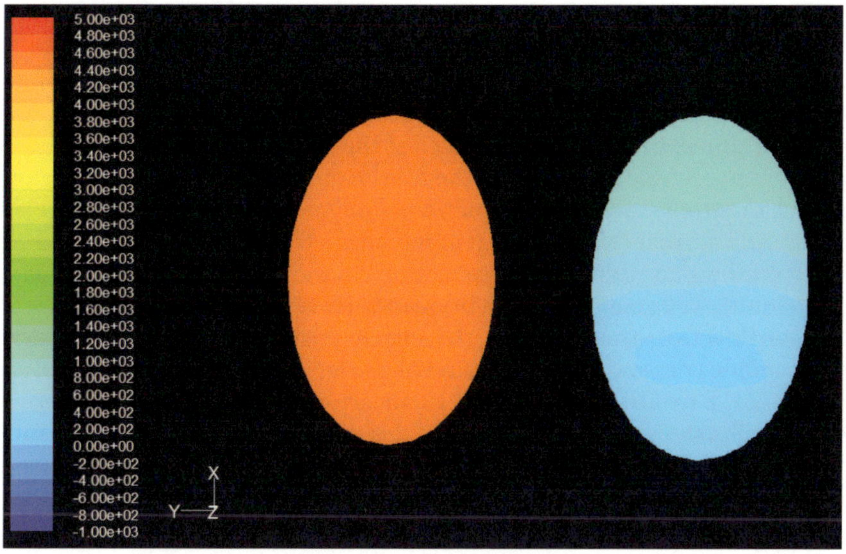


**Figure 10.**
*Comparison of the pressure before (left) and after (right) the stenosis (note: For a better illustration of the pressure gradient over the cross section, the top and bottom values of the scale have changed).*

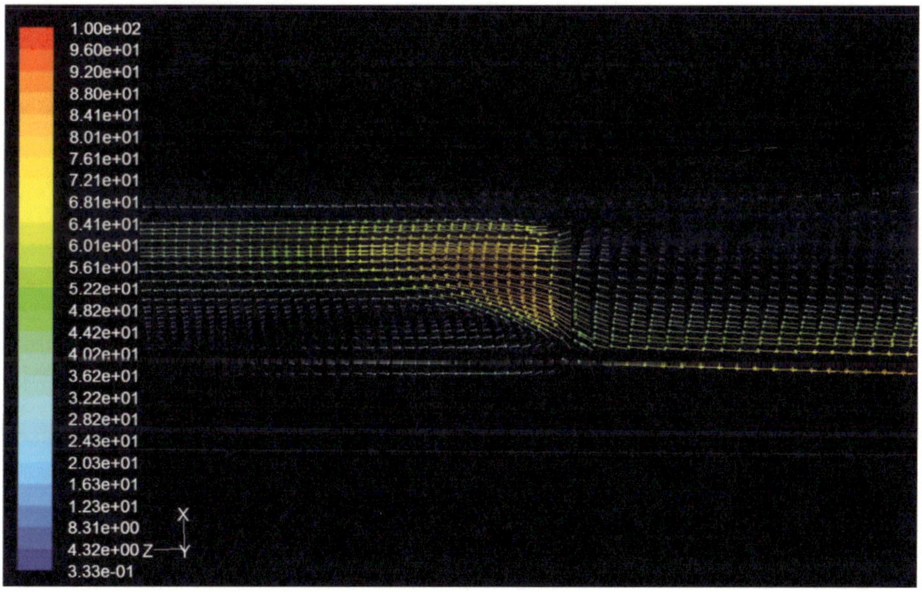


**Figure 11.**
*Backflows both before (top right) and after (bottom left) the stenosis.*

## 4. Discussion

When reflecting on currents in tubes with round cross sections, a laminar airflow with parabolic velocity profile primarily springs to mind [13]. The current can present itself in a completely different matter and is illustrated by the airflow dynamics of the laryngoscope. Unique current patterns and pressure dynamics are created due to the technical specifications of the laryngoscope. Although the jet ventilation technique is a recognized and widely used method of jet ventilation technique [14, 15], no data on airflow and pressure dynamics have been published to date. As shown by the data, both gas nozzles emit gas with the characteristics of a free jet [16, 17]. The free jet involving friction [18] then undergoes the typical expansion of the jet. While the nozzle produces a high entrance velocity, the velocity drops downstream due to energy loss of the projected fluid beam because of friction with the surrounding fluid. An entrainment [19] of air is induced at the edges of the laryngoscope due to the big difference in velocity between the free beam and the fluid in the laryngoscope. This, in turn, results in the reduction of oxygen by room air. Nevertheless, our results indicate that this entrainment includes a fraction of the projected gas, so that we could show an additional recirculation component of the projected gas when utilizing simultaneous high- and low-frequency jet ventilation. The lower the acceleration of airflow from the nozzles is, the smaller entrainment could be measured. These phenomena depend on the pressure of the jet gas, the gas velocity [20], and as Koller et al. [21] have already shown the localization of the jet nozzles.

As our results show, the gas flow can be described as asymmetrical and simultaneous bidirectional. The asymmetry is caused by the positioning of the jet nozzles. On the side of the nozzles, the jet gas flows in the direction of lungs with a high z-axis velocity. Even though the primary velocity of the emitted gas at the nozzle can be as high as 300 m/s, it reduces speed to 70 m/s at the tip of the endoscope. Because the velocity is only very high at the nozzle exit, it is acceptable to observe the common respiratory gases as incompressible fluids [22]. The term simultaneous bidirectional describes the synchronically process of gas transfer into the lung and from the lung by the continuous high-frequency jet ventilation. The low-frequency gas application takes place discontinuously.

### 4.1 Stenosis

The clinically relevant scenario of laryngeal or subglottic stenosis and obvious reduction of ventilation diameter (stenosis) is found at the tip of the endoscope. In contrast to previously publicized studies, which assume the nozzles of jet ventilation lie in close proximity to the tip of the endoscope [23], our supraglottic jet ventilation model uses the clinically accurate gas release point, located more proximally. Therefore, presuming that the previously published data is based on a gas release point of 1 cm proximal to the endoscope tip, this data is an incomparable data based on a proximal release point for supraglottic jet ventilation, which lies 6–8 cm proximally to the endoscope tip. Additionally, the pre-stenotic pressure plays an essential role in the gas passage through the stenotic pathology. It is not surprising that, as our results indicate, the pre-stenotic pressure drastically rises, while the velocity drops. The reduction in diameter is however also responsible for the increase in localized back draft and reduced entrainment. As we could show, there is also a pressure drop within the stenosis, which is also pronounced immediately after passage through the stenosis and continues for a finite distance post-stenotically. The fact that the pre-stenotic pressure is high and low in the post-stenotic area is not surprising from a fluid mechanical view. Our results show that in our case, the gas velocity drops pre-stenotically, just to rise again within the stenosis, only to drop again after the stenosis. The results demonstrate that the pressure during inspiration is higher in front of the stenosis than after the stenosis. Since stenosis represents an abrupt cross-sectional constriction, the Bernoulli equation may be included in fluid mechanical considerations only in enlargement by an operating element and pressure loss coefficient [24, 25]. Even though this physical law is widely known, many physicians and surgeons are unaware of its implication for laryngeal stenosis and often assume pressure to be higher post-stenotically [26].

## 5. Conclusion

Our results imply that if sole high-frequency gas dynamics can be compared to steady flow, then additional low-frequency gas flow should be seen as unsteady flow. It would be recommendable to investigate the transient case and add a user-defined function (UDF) to the calculation program to better understand and examine the gas flow within the laryngoscope. This notwithstanding, our data sheds new light on the flow patterns and dynamics of applied gas in the endoscope and contributes to a better understanding of jet ventilation as ventilation technique. This is especially true for the clinically highly relevant stenotic airway.

## 6. Respiratory devices

A new respiratory device (TwinStream, Carl Reiner, Vienna, Austria) has been developed for superimposed high-frequency jet ventilation (SHFJV) (**Figure 12**). Although the new technique is successfully used in clinical studies [27], there are few explanations about the structure and mechanism of the respirator. It is designed to allow both low-frequency and high-frequency jet ventilations simultaneously. An upper (plateau) and lower (positive end-expiratory pressure (PEEP) should be formed (**Figure 13**). The effectiveness of this combination causes an increased efficiency of gas exchange [28–30]. In addition, the ratio of inspiratory duration and expiratory duration (I/E ratio) can be determined. In contrast to previously used proportional valves, four matrix valves are used each. The gas of the central gas supply is mixed in the chambers—an algorithm recognizes the demand from the consumption (emission pressure, frequency, and I/E ratio) as well as the necessary oxygen mixture. Four matrix valves per medium (O2 and compressed air) tailed depending on the requirements and thus ensure the exact mixture. The chambers also allow intermediate storage and ensure that the gas output is constant and changes when the oxygen concentration changes.

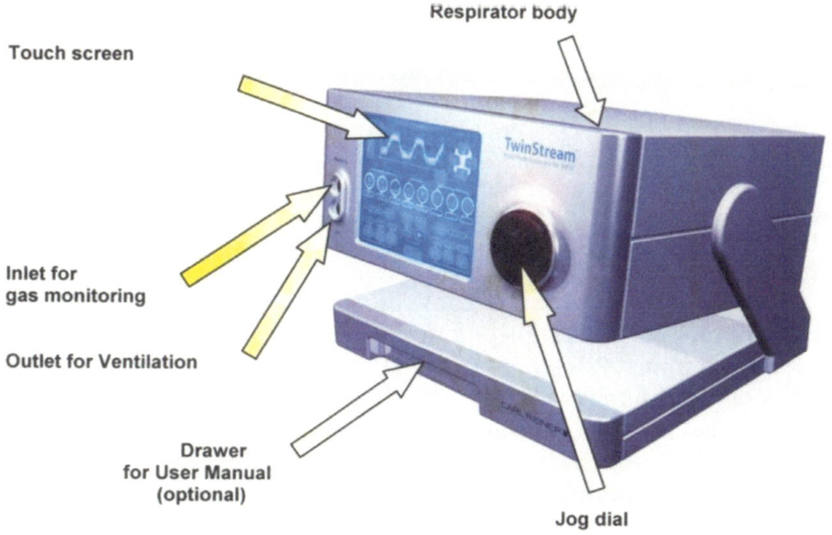


**Figure 12.**
*Jet respirator (TwinStream).*

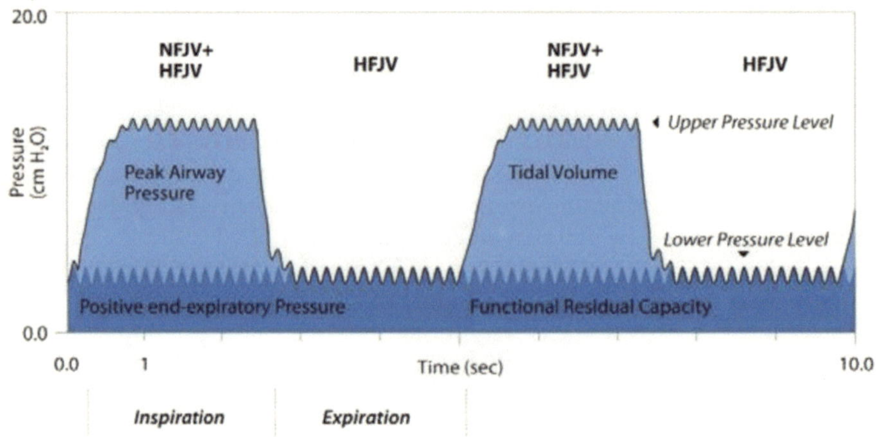


**Figure 13.**
*Inspiration and expiration during SHFJV, NFJV – Normofrequent Jet Ventilation; HFJV – High Frequency Jet Ventilation.*

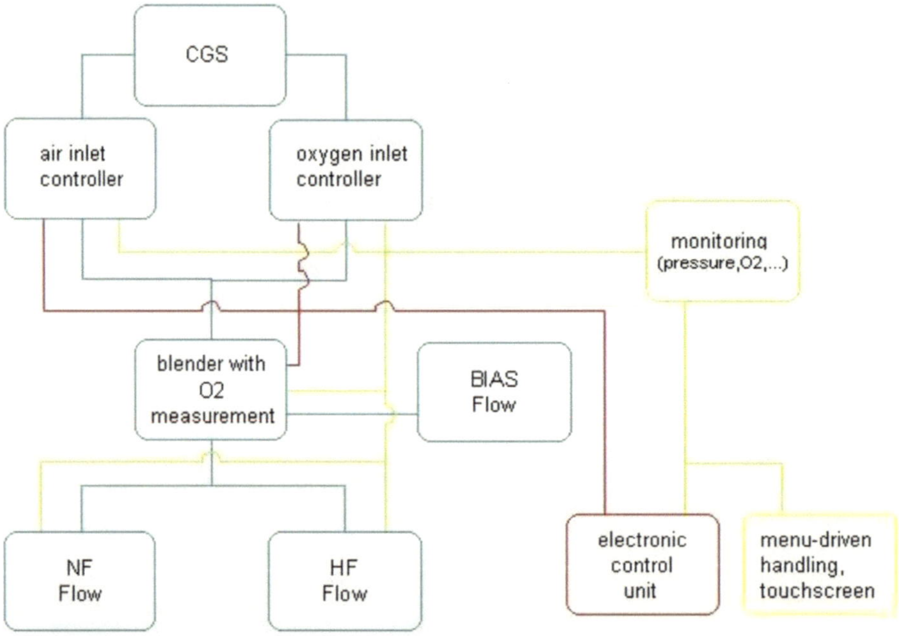


**Figure 14.**
*Respirator (TwinStream) pneumatic diagram.*

The advantages of the matrix valves are the shortest switching times, no friction losses, and trouble-free generation of high frequencies. All parameters are controlled via a programmable logic controller (PLC). The frequencies and pressures that can be used in different ways have significantly extended the spectrum of the respiratory device. Since the gas coming from the nozzles is not humidified and warmed up, an additional gas flow is added to this gas (bias flow). This gas is heated and humidified by a humidifier (**Figure 14**).

In addition to its operational application, it can thus also be used in the intensive care with a jet modifier.

The superimposed high-frequency ventilation (SHFJV) respirator is flow-variable, time-controlled, and pressure-controlled ventilation. This form of jet ventilation is closest to the conventional form of biphasic positive airway pressure ventilation. But it is a pulsatile ventilation. The low-frequency jet ventilation (NFJV) unit generates the upper pressure plateau during the inspiration phase (PIP—peak pressure). The high-frequency jet ventilation (HFJV) unit runs continuously and generates the lower-pressure plateau—positive end-expiratory pressure (PEEP).

The TwinStream jet ventilation system was developed for artificial ventilation of patients under anesthesia during diagnostic and surgical interventions in the

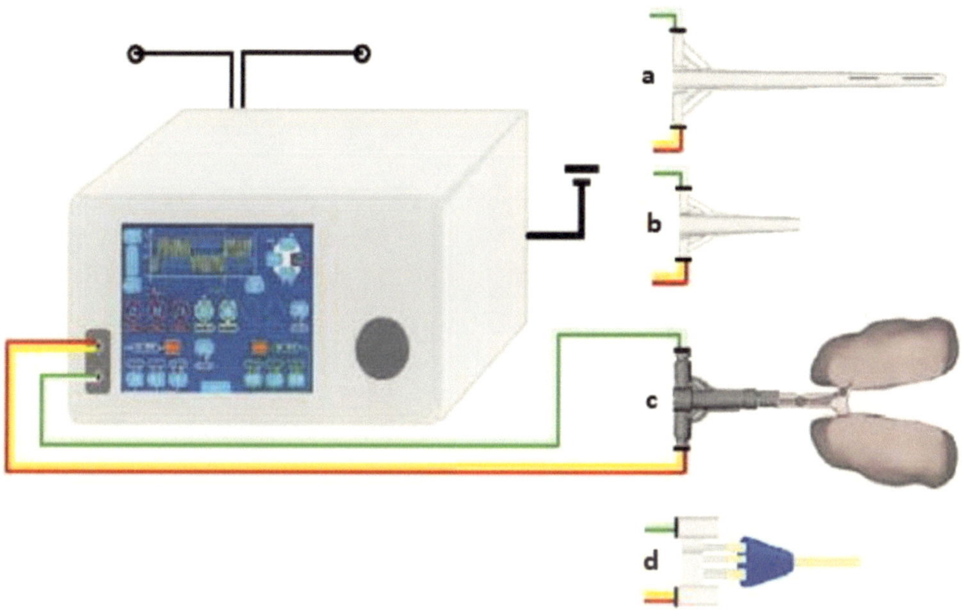


**Figure 15.**
*TwinStream connection diagram for use with jet instrument rigid bronchoscope (a), jet instrument rigid laryngoscope (b), jet converter (c) that allows continuous ventilation through an endotracheal tube or a laryngeal mask, and jet catheter (d) which can also be used for ventilation.*

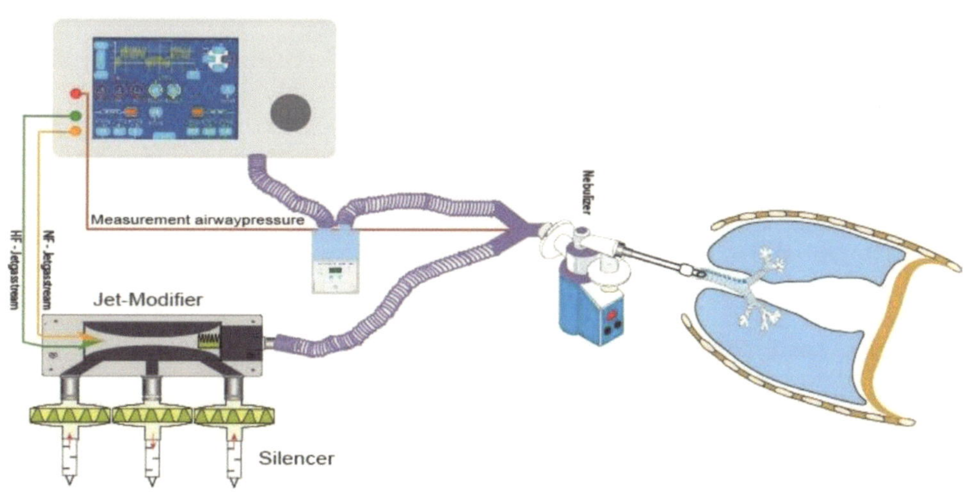


**Figure 16.**
*Connection schematic for the use in the intensive care.*

entire respiratory system. This ventilation system, with its special accessories and jet catheters, is appropriate for thoracic surgical use such as resection of the trachea (**Figure 15**). First, results show that this respirator is suitable for the treatment in patients with ARDS, lung fistulas, or multiple trauma at the intensive care unit. This advanced application requires a jet modifier (**Figure 16**). In this jet modifier, the superposition of the jet gas and its transport during the inspiration into the lungs as well as the gas outflow in the expiration phase take place.

In addition to jet ventilation, there is application of high-frequency oscillation in intensive care medicine [31, 32]. It is a recognized procedure. If small tidal volumes are emitted from a nozzle during jet ventilation, the tidal volumes are generated and transported at the high-frequency oscillation by vibrations of a membrane with a high frequency. Both techniques lead to an improvement in gas exchange. For a long time, it was believed that this improvement was due to increased diffusion mechanisms. Improved radiological techniques, however, show that they are due to a recruitment of alveoli.

## Author details

Alexander Aloy[1], Simon Hell[1], Andreas Nowak[2]* and Matthaeus Grasl[3]

1 University of Technology Vienna, Institute of Fluid Mechanics and Heat Transfer, Vienna, Austria

2 Department of Anesthesiology and Intensive Care Medicine, Emergency and Pain Medicine, Hospital Dresden, Friedrichstadt, Germany

3 Department of Ear, Nose and Throat Diseases, Medical University of Vienna, Vienna Austria

*Address all correspondence to: alexander@aloy.at

## References

[1] Andersson B, Andersson R. Computational Fluid Dynamics for Engineers. Göteborg, Sweden: Cambridge University Press; 2011

[2] Yin Y, Ci J, Hoffmann EA, Tawhai MH, Lin C-L. Simulation of pulmonary air flow with a subject-specific boundary condition. Journal of Biomechanical Engineering. 2010;**43**:2159-2163

[3] Walters DK, Luke WH. Computational fluid dynamics simulations of particle deposition in large-scale, multigenerational lung models. Journal of Biomechanical Engineering. 2011;**133**(1). 8 pages

[4] Calkins JM, Waterson CK, Hameroff SR, Kanel J. Jet pulse characteristic for high-frequency jet ventilation in dogs. Anesthesia and Analgesia. 1982;**61**:293-300

[5] Orloff LA, Parhizkar N, Ortiz E. The Hunsaker Mon-jet ventilation tube for microlaryngeal surgery: Optimal laryngeal exposure. Ear, Nose, & Throat Journal. 2002;**81**:390-394

[6] Bourgain JL, Desruennes E, Fischler M, Ravussin P. Transtracheal high frequency jet ventilation for endoscopic airway surgery: A multicenter study. British Journal of Anaesthesia. 2001;**87**:870-875

[7] Barakate M, Maver E, Wotherspoon G, Havas T. Anaesthesia for microlaryngeal and laser laryngeal surgery: Impact of subglottic jet ventilation. The Journal of Laryngology and Otology. 2010;**124**:641-645

[8] Aloy A, Schachner M, Cancura W. Tubeless translaryngeal superimposed jet ventilation. European Archives of Oto-Rhino-Laryngology. 1991;**248**:475-478

[9] Sigloch H. Technische Fluidmechanik. Springer Dordrecht Heidelberg London NewYork: Springer Verlag; 2011

[10] Aloy A, Kimla T, Schrag E, Donner A, Grasl M. Tubuslose superponierte Hochfrequenz-Jet-Ventilation (SHFJV) bei hochgradigen laryngealen Stenosen. Laryngo-Rhino-Otol. 1994;**73**:405-411

[11] Depirerraz B, Ravussin P, Brossad E, Monnier P. Percutaneous transtracheal jet ventilation for paediatric endoscopic laser treatment of laryngeal and subglottic lesions. Canadian Journal of Anaesthesia. 1995;**42**:554-556

[12] Rezaie-Majd A, Bigenzahn W, Denk D-M, Burian M, Kornfehl J, Grasl MC, et al. Superimposed high-frequency jet ventilation (SHFJV) for endoscopic laryngotracheal surgery in more than 1500 patients. British Journal of Anaesthesia. 2006;**96**:650-659

[13] Surek D, Stempin S. Angewandte Strömungsmechanik für Praxis und Studium. Wiesbaden Germany: Teubner Verlag/GWV Fachverlage GmbH; 2007

[14] Aloy A, Schachner M, Cancura W. Tubuslose translaryngeale superponierte jet-ventilation. Der Anaesthesist. 1990;**39**:493-498

[15] Friedrich G, Mausser G, Gugatschka M. Die Jet-Ventilation in der operativen Laryngologie. HNO. 2008;**12**:1197-1206

[16] Schobeiri MT. Fluid Mechanics for Engineers: A Graduate Textbook. Berlin Heidelberg: Springer Verlag; 2010

[17] Durst F. Grundlagen der Strömungsmechanik: Eine Einführung in die Theorie der Strömungen von Fluiden. Berlin Heidelberg New York: Springer Verlag; 2006

[18] Schade H, Kunz E. *Strömungslehre*. Berlin: de Gruyter Verlag; 2007

[19] Pijush K, Ira MC. *Fluid Mechanics*. London Wall: Academic Press sn imprint of Elsevier; 2010

[20] Falcone AM, Cataldo JC. Entrainment velocity in an axisymmetric turbulent jet. Journal of Fluids Engineering. 2003;**125**(4):620-627

[21] Koller-Milosevic D, Schneider W. Free and confined jets at low Reynolds numbers. Fluid Dynamic Research. 1993;**12**(6):307-327

[22] Siekmann HE. Strömungslehre: Grundlagen. Berlin Heidelberg: Springer Verlag; 2000

[23] Ng A, Russell WC, Harvey N, Thompson JP. Comparing methods of high frequency jet ventilation in a model of Laryngotracheal stenosis. Anest Analg. 2002;**95**:764-769

[24] Kuhlmann HC. Strömungsmechanik. ein Imprint von Pearson Education München/Germany. Boston. San Francisco. Harlow, England: Paerson Studium; 2007

[25] Böswirth L, Bschorer S. Technische Strömungslehre: Lehr- und Übungsbuch. Springer Fachmedien Wiesbaden GmbH Germany: Vieweg u. Teubner; 2012

[26] Buczkowski PW, Fombon FN, Lin ES, Russsel WC, Thompson JP. Air entrainment during high-frequency jet ventilation in a model of upper tracheal stenosis. British Journal of Anesthesia. 2007;**99**:891-897

[27] Hohenforst-Schmidt W, Zarogoulidis P, Huang H, Man YG, Laskou S, Koulouris C, et al. A new and safe mode of ventilation for interventional pulmonary medicine: The ease of nasal superimposed high frequency jet ventilation. Journal of Cancer. 2018;**9**(5):816-833

[28] R S, LoMauro A, Gandolfi S, Priori R, Aliverti A, Frykholm P, et al. Influence of tracheal obstruction on the efficacy of superimposed high-frequency jet ventilation and single-frequency jet ventilation. Anesthesiology. 2015;**123**(4):799-909

[29] Jiang Y, Kacmarek RM. Efficacy of superimposed high-frequency jet ventilation applied to variable degrees of tracheal stenosis: One step forward to optimized patient care. Anesthesiology. 2015;**123**:747-749

[30] Putz L, Mayne A, Dincq. Jet ventilation during rigid bronchoscopy in adults: A focused review. Bio Med Research InternationaI. 2016. Article ID 4234861, 6 pages

[31] Xu-Xiong G, Zhao-Ni W, Ya-Ting L, Li P, Li-Fen Y, Yan H, Yue-Yu S, Liang-Ming C, Zhuang-Gui C. High-frequency oscillatory ventilation is an effective treatment for severe pediatric acute respiratory distress syndrome with refractory hypoxemia. Therapeutics and Clinical Risk Management. 2016;**12**:1563-1571

[32] Chang HK. Mechanism of gas transport during ventilation by high-frequency oscillation. Journal of Applied Physiology: Respiratory, Environmental and Exercise Physiology. Mar 1984;**56**(3):653-663

Section 3

# Rehabilitation

Chapter 3

# Application of a Robotic Rehabilitation Training System for Recovery of Severe Plegie Hand Motor Function after a Stroke

*Hirofumi Tanabe, Munehiro Ikuta, Toshimasa Mikawa, Akihiko Kondo and Yoshifumi Morita*

## Abstract

We have developed a rehabilitation training system (UR-System-PARKO: Useful and Ultimate Rehabilitation System-PARKO) for patients after a stroke to promote recovery of motor function of the severe plegic hand with hemiplegia. A clinical test with six patients for the therapeutic effect of the UR-System-PARKO for severe plegic hand was performed. For all patients, the active ranges of motion (total active motion) of finger extension improved after training with the UR-System-PARKO. Moreover, the modified Ashworth scale (MAS) scores of finger extension increased. Thus, the training reduced the spastic paralysis. These results suggest the effectiveness of training with the UR-System-PARKO for recovery of motor function as defined by finger extension in the severe plegic hand.

**Keywords:** stroke, hemiplegia, finger, rehabilitation device, motor recovery

## 1. Introduction

Stroke is the leading cause of disability in Japan, with more than 1 million people in Japan living with a disability as a result of stroke. Therefore, interventions that address the sensorimotor impairments resulting from stroke are important. Motor function may be restored more than 6 months after a stroke [1, 2], but these studies included patients with only moderate poststroke hemiplegia, whereas most stroke survivors have a severely plegic hand with difficulty extending the fingers [3]. This suggests that a method is needed for treatment of these severely affected cases. However, although a few studies on rehabilitation therapy for severe plegic hands have been reported, no marked recovery of ability in extension of the fingers of the plegic hands was achieved in any study [4, 5]. Proprioceptive neuromuscular facilitation (PNF) is a therapeutic method that was reported to increase the muscle strength of the plegic extremities in patients with stroke-induced hemiplegia [6]. However, since PNF is indicated for patients with a certain level of joint motion, this method has not been used for severe plegic hands where the fingers cannot extend. Thus, the first author developed a method to build up the extensor digitorum muscle strength using PNF [7, 8] for stroke patients with severe hemiplegia.

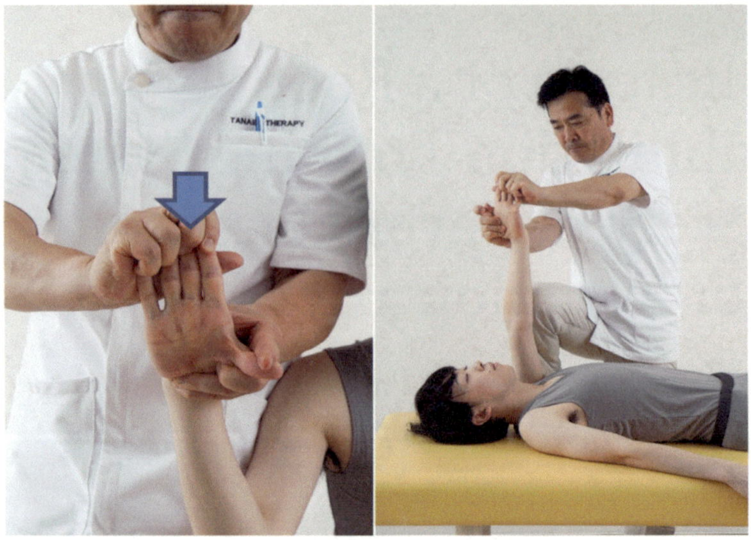


**Figure 1.**
*The first author has developed the TANABE therapy for severe hemiplegic stroke patients.*

With this therapy, he has performed repeated facilitation training using his hands on stroke patients with a severe plegic hand to help them recover their motor function, and a good treatment outcome was achieved [9, 10] (**Figure 1**).

Facilitation training uses extension of the elbow joint with resistance applied to the tips of the fully extended hemiplegic fingers to increase the force of the extensor digitorum muscle. However, this approach is time-consuming for the therapist. Therefore, development of a training system is required instead of repeated facilitation training by a therapist. The objectives of this study were to develop a training system to increase the output of the extensor digitorum muscle force and to verify the effect of training with the developed system on a severe plegic hand. The training system is called the UR-System-PARKO (a useful and ultimate rehabilitation support system for PARKO). The UR-System-PARKO was developed by remodeling the simplified training system, which developed previously for resistance training of hemiplegic upper limbs [11]. A brace for securing the plegic hand to the UR-System-PARKO was developed on the basis of repeated facilitation training by a therapist.

## 2. Facilitation training for finger extension

Facilitation training is indicated for patients with severely plegic hands who cannot extend their fingers. The training increases the extensor digitorum muscle force, and finger extension can be achieved with 2–3 min of manual training by a therapist. However, to retain the effect until the following day, training should be performed for at least 1 h a day, and manual facilitation training by a therapist is demanding work. However, since all of the interphalangeal finger joints should be totally maintained in the full extension position with a certain level of resistance during the facilitation training, the maximum duration of the training provided by a therapist with no break is about 10 min. Although the details of the operating procedures of the facilitation training will be explained later, several therapists will be required to provide this manual facilitation training for 1 h or more on a rotating basis. Thus, a very aggressive intervention is needed and will involve robotization of the training.

### 2.1 Plegic hand fingers always bend

Human fingers are constructed so as to prioritize flexion to extension movement in order to grab objects. Thus, fingers are lightly bent, even at rest. After a stroke, the upper limb and fingers on the plegic side are usually controlled by synkinesis of the flexor muscles, and this often results in clenching of the fingers. Our hypothesis is that contraction of the muscle for extending the fingers (extensor digitorum) is inhibited by strong contraction of muscles bending the fingers (flexor digitorum profundus, flexor digitorum superficialis) in severely plegic hands. We have found that contraction of the flexor muscles is inhibited and that of the extensor muscle is induced by fixing all fingers in a hyperextended position and extending the elbow joint while applying resistance to the fingertips. The reason why the plegic hand fingers are able to extend under these two conditions is explained below.

### 2.2 Why are severe plegic hands unable to open?

a. Flexor and extensor muscles are present in pairs in the joints. For joint movement, neither the flexor nor the extensor muscle contract alone, but both contract simultaneously, giving smooth and accurate movement. The balance of the two muscles in joint movement is not 0 vs. 100%, but about 46 vs. 54% or 44 vs. 56%, and the slight dominance of either muscle again results in smooth movement [12]. However, in poststroke plegic hands, the flexor muscle tone is excessive and the finger flexor muscle contracts more strongly than the extensor muscle. Therefore, as a plegic hand is opened to grasp objects, the appropriate balance of the two muscles is not present. This inability to grasp objects is due to the stronger contraction of the flexor muscles, which results in strong hand clenching.

b. Marked extensor digitorum muscle contraction is induced by fixation of the plegic hand in a hyperextended position, and this contraction is further increased by extending the plegic hand forward while applying resistance to the fingertips of this hand. Hogan stated that simultaneous contraction increases stiffness of the joint and maintains the position of the plegic hand [13]. Muscle spindles that sense the muscle length are adjusted by $\gamma$ motor neurons. The length of the flexor muscles gradually shortens as finger flexion is induced by contraction of these muscles, but simultaneous actions of $\alpha$ and $\gamma$ motor neurons prevent sensitivity reduction of muscle spindles ($\alpha$-$\gamma$ linkage). When the fingertips push an object with the fingers fixed and extended, the flexor and extensor muscles contract simultaneously to stabilize the joint. The muscles cancel out the tension on each other, and there is no change in muscle length, while the $\alpha$-$\gamma$ linkage prevents a change in muscle spindle sensitivity. Thus, muscle spindle sensitivity is increased by afferent contraction compared with that in muscle shortening, which increases the roles of the finger flexor and extensor muscles in the stretch reflex. The flexion activity of the hyperextended fingers is reduced, despite the contraction of the finger flexor muscles. In contrast, this contraction easily extends the fingers, resulting in marked contraction of the finger extensor muscle (**Figure 2**).

Additional resistance applied to the fingertips increases the output of the finger extensor muscle force. The flexion/extension torque of the interphalangeal joint varies depending on the finger joint angle, despite the similar forces of the flexor and extensor muscles of the fingers. This position is significant for flexion movement (**Figure 2a**). The torque of joint rotation in the extension direction decreases because the extensor digitorum muscle tendon is in contact with the bone. Conversely, the torque of rotation in the flexion direction increases because

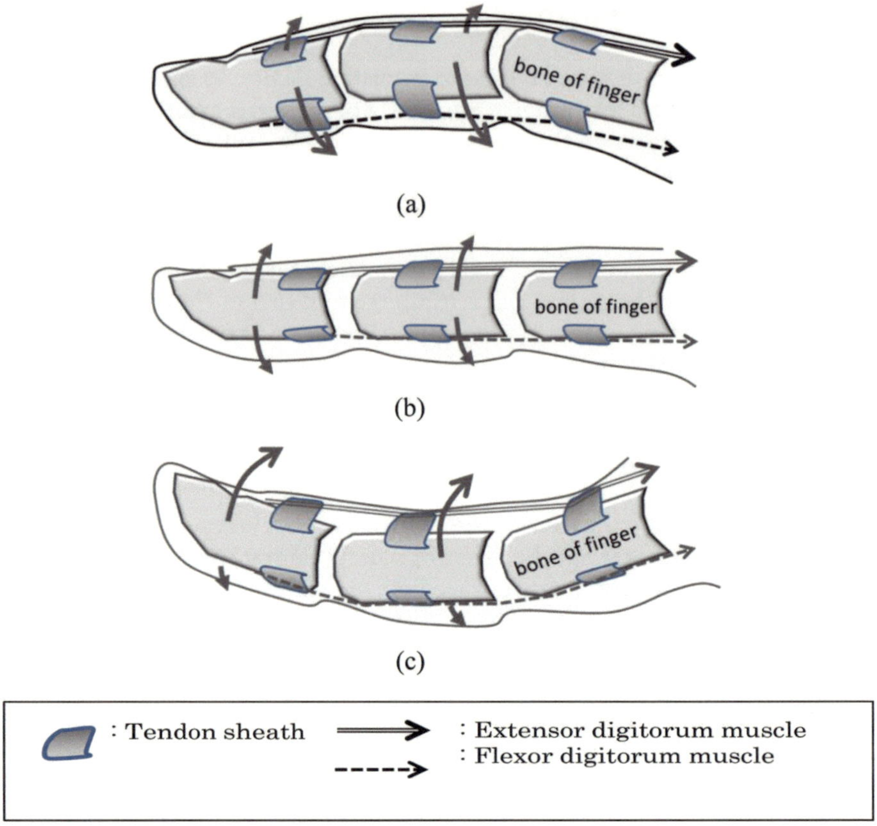


**Figure 2.**
*Differences in the torque of joint movement in finger extension and flexion between the flexor and extensor muscles of the fingers. (a) Position with light flexion of the finger; (b) position with extension of the finger; and (c) position with hyperextension of the finger.*

the flexor digitorum muscle tendon acts to pull the tendon sheath away from the bone. The torques of rotation of the interphalangeal joint in the flexion/extension direction of the flexor and in the extensor muscles are the same (**Figure 2b**) and this position is significant for extension movement (**Figure 2c**). The torque of joint rotation in the extension direction increases because the extensor digitorum muscle tendon pulls the tendon sheath away from the bone. Simultaneous contraction in joints increases stiffness and muscle spindle sensitivity and thus may increase the gain of the stretch reflex loop. The extensor muscle-dominant increase in output occurs because the range of motion of the fingers is greater in the flexion direction because the fingers easily bend under an external force against which output of the extensor muscle force may increase to boost stiffness.

## 3. Training system for recovery of motor function

The training system consists of a force display system with rotational system of one degree-of-freedom and a brace for securing the paralyzed hand. The force display system was developed in our previous work [14, 15]. The brace was developed in this work. The training system was named the UR-System-PARKO, which is shown in **Figure 3**. In order to satisfy the conditions (1) and (2) to facilitate finger extension, the force display system was used and a new brace was developed, respectively.

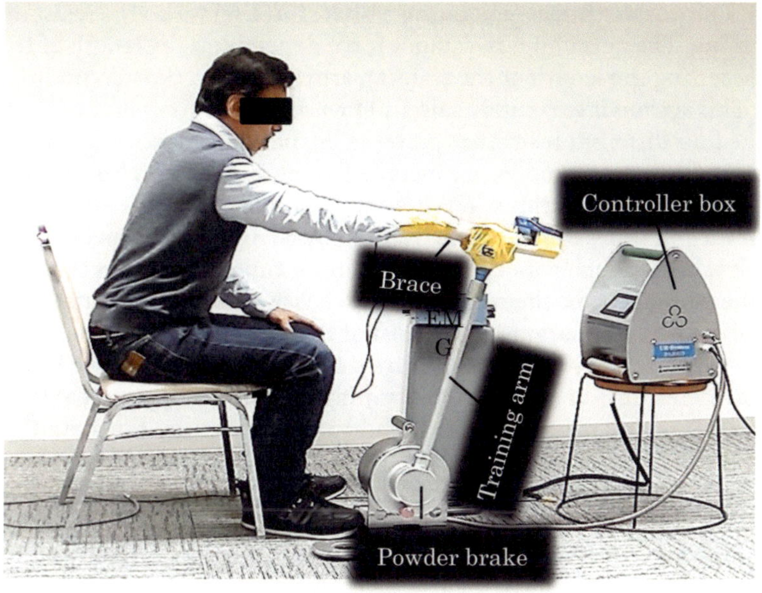


(a)

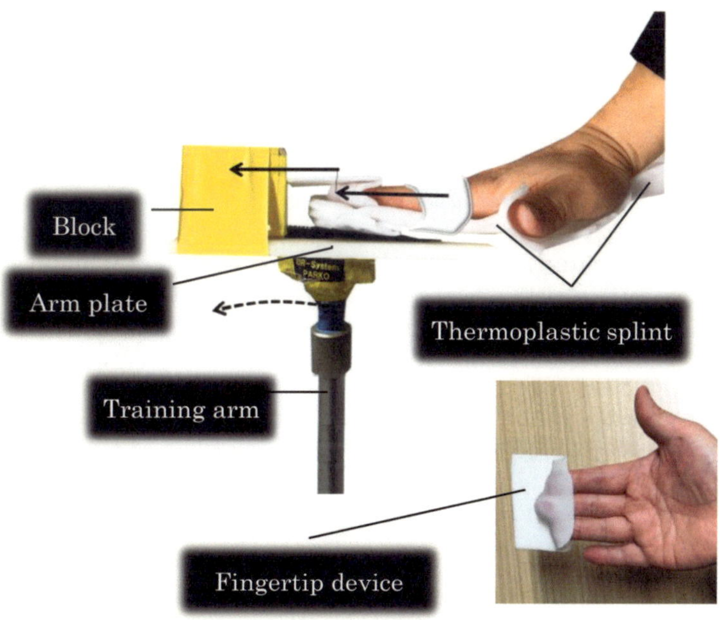


(b)

**Figure 3.**
*UR-System PARKO. (a) Whole system and (b) brace.*

### 3.1 Force display system

The force display system has a mechanical system and a controller. The mechanical system consists of a training arm and a powder brake (SINFONIA TECHNOLOGY CO., Ltd., PRB-2.5H). The brace attached to the tip of the training arm is used to secure the patient's hand to the apparatus. The patient moves the brace forward and backward by himself/herself while stretching and bending the elbow repeatedly. The powder brake generating a brake force serves as the resistance force during training. The maximum resistance force depends on the length of the training arm. When setting the length of the training arm to 0.75 m, the maximum resistance was 49 N. This system is extremely safe and low cost, because it is not equipped with motors. The four different resistance patterns, namely a step mode, a slope mode, a wall mode, and a constant mode, are installed in the controller. This system is mainly equipped with the two functions. The resistance display function enables therapists to perform various types of resistance training by changing the arm length and the resistance level. The touch panel parameter setting function enables therapists to easily set the parameters of the resistance patterns by pushing the buttons on the touch panel display. The parameters consist of the magnitudes and the positions of the resistance patterns. The magnitudes are selected from among nine levels. The positions are determined by moving the training arm and stopping it at the desired position. This function provides good visibility and ease of use for therapists.

### 3.2 Brace to facilitate finger extension

A new brace was developed to facilitate finger extension, which is shown in **Figure 3b**. The brace consists of an arm plate, a thermoplastic splint, a fingertip device, and a block. The arm plate was fixed to the tip of the training arm with flexibility. The block was fixed on the arm plate. The thermoplastic splint was made to fix the plegic hand of a hemiplegic patient in complete extension. The fingertip device attaching to the second to fourth fingers was made of a thermoplastic plate. Since the fingertip device is the important part for acting the equal resistance force to the three finger tips, it was prepared for each subject. Since contraction of the fifth finger extensor muscle is improved with facilitation of contraction of the extensor digitorum muscles of the second to fourth fingers, the fifth finger was not attached to the fingertip device. Since the fingertip device is slightly movable in the direction of travel on the rail on the arm plate, the force acting on the fingertip device moves the training arm. The movable range was 1 mm. This means that the point of action to resistance force generated by the UR-System-PARKO is the contact point between the fingertip device and the block.

## 4. Clinical evaluation of therapeutic effect

We conducted clinical tests of intensive training with the UR-System PARKO for severely affected hands with little or no extension of the wrist, fingers, and thumb.

### 4.1 Participants

The participants were six patients with chronic hemiplegia after stroke who were admitted to the clinic between September 2017 and July 2018 (**Table 1**). Before training, all participants could not extend the fingers and thumb and grasp and release the items.

### 4.2 Methods

All participants conducted intensive training using the UR-System-PARKO for 2 h/day and 2 weeks. The participants were requested to perform the intensive training using the UR-System-PARKO at their own pace. After each set (50 times) of the training, they took a rest for 10 min, with their hands withdrawn from the UR-System-PARKO. It took about 4–4.5 min to complete one set of the training. All participants performed the training for about eight sets. After the fourth set, they rested for 30 min, and a therapist stretched and massaged the upper extremities and fingers.

| Subject | Gender | Age | Hemiplegia | Handedness | Poststroke (year) |
|---|---|---|---|---|---|
| Subject 1 | M | 51 | L | R | 8 |
| Subject 2 | M | 66 | L | R | 2 |
| Subject 3 | F | 53 | L | R | 2 |
| Subject 4 | M | 70 | R | R | 4 |
| Subject 5 | F | 45 | L | R | 3 |
| Subject 6 | M | 43 | R | R | 3 |

*Note: M = male, F = female, R = right, L = left.*

**Table 1.**
*Participant demographic data.*

| Subject | | TAM (deg) | | % TAM | |
|---|---|---|---|---|---|
| | | Pre | Post | Pre | Post |
| Subject 1 | Index finger | 5 | 50 | 2 | 19 |
| | Middle finger | 5 | 75 | 2 | 29 |
| | Ring finger | 0 | 55 | 0 | 21 |
| | Little finger | 0 | 60 | 0 | 23 |
| | Total | 10 | 240 | 0.0 | 0.9 |
| Subject 2 | Index finger | 5 | 90 | 2 | 35 |
| | Middle finger | 0 | 45 | 0 | 17 |
| | Ring finger | 0 | 45 | 0 | 17 |
| | Little finger | 0 | 30 | 0 | 12 |
| | Total | 5 | 210 | 0.0 | 0.8 |
| Subject 3 | Index finger | 5 | 50 | 2 | 19 |
| | Middle finger | 5 | 75 | 2 | 29 |
| | Ring finger | 0 | 55 | 0 | 21 |
| | Little finger | 0 | 60 | 0 | 23 |
| | Total | 10 | 240 | 0.0 | 0.9 |
| Subject 4 | Index finger | 15 | 120 | 6 | 46 |
| | Middle finger | 10 | 135 | 4 | 52 |
| | Ring finger | 0 | 90 | 0 | 35 |
| | Little finger | 0 | 80 | 0 | 31 |
| | Total | 25 | 425 | 0.1 | 1.6 |
| Subject 5 | Index finger | 0 | 35 | 0 | 13 |
| | Middle finger | 0 | 20 | 0 | 8 |
| | Ring finger | 0 | 10 | 0 | 4 |
| | Little finger | 0 | 10 | 0 | 4 |
| | Total | 0 | 75 | 0.0 | 0.3 |
| Subject 6 | Index finger | 5 | 110 | 2 | 42 |
| | Middle finger | 5 | 140 | 2 | 54 |
| | Ring finger | 0 | 40 | 0 | 15 |
| | Little finger | 0 | 35 | 0 | 13 |
| | Total | 10 | 325 | 0.0 | 1.3 |

*Pre: before intensive training; post: after intensive training; change: difference between the results before and after training.*

**Table 2.**
*TAM and % TAM scores before and after 2-week intensive training with the UR-System-PARKO.*

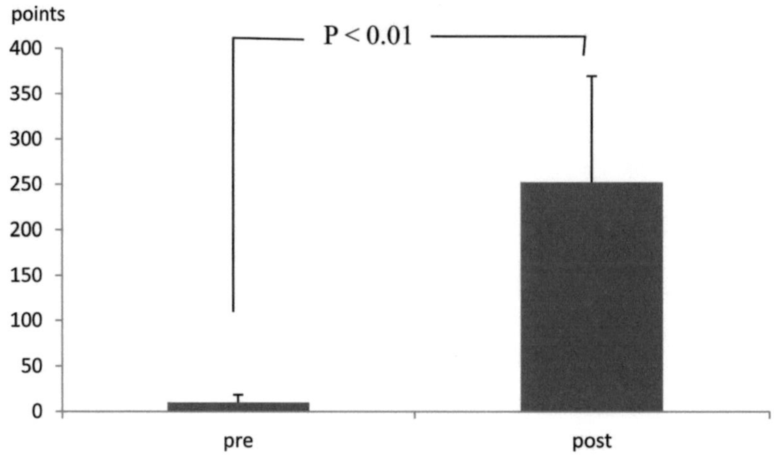


**Figure 4.**
*TAM scores before and after 2-week intensive training with the UR-System-PARKO.*

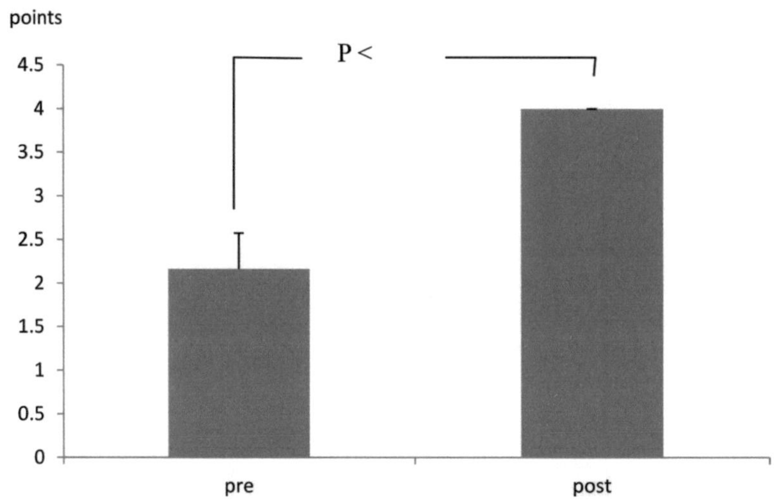


**Figure 5.**
*MAS scores before and after 2-week intensive training with the UR-System-PARKO.*

### 4.3 Assessment

The therapeutic effect before and after intensive training was assessed using the Total Active Motion (TAM) and modified Ashworth scale (MAS). TAM describes the full arc of motion of the digits and is measured as the total flexion of the three finger joints minus the loss of full extension of these joints: TAM = (metacarpophalangeal [MP] + proximal interphalangeal [PIP] + distal interphalangeal [DIP] flexion)−(MP + PIP + DIP extension loss). TAM was measured before the 2-week intensive training and on the day after the last day of training.

### 4.4 Results

All participants underwent intense intensive training according to the predetermined protocol. The TAM score for upper extremity motion showed significant improvement for participants (**Table 2, Figure 4**). Post hoc analysis indicated significant differences between pre- and posttreatment scores, and the mean TAM scores increased by 0.003 ($P < 0.01$), respectively. The MAS scores showed a significant attenuation effect on spasticity, with post hoc analysis revealing significant differences between pre- and posttreatment scores increased by 0.001 ($P < 0.05$, **Figure 5**). The results of the study suggest that intense intensive training for severely affected hands with little or no extension of the fingers and thumbs improves the functions of the affected-side upper extremity.

## 5. Conclusions

The therapeutic effect of the training with the UR-System-PARKO was shown. It was found that induction of contraction of the extensor digitorum muscle of plegic hands required the following two conditions: "hyperextension of all fingers" and "extension movement of the elbow joint while applying resistance load to the finger tips." In the clinical study with the 2-week intensive training, the motor function of the paralyzed hand was improved, and the spasticity of the flexor muscle was decreased. As a manual technique to facilitate the movement of plegic limbs of poststroke hemiplegia patients, Kabat et al. developed Proprioceptive Neuromuscular Facilitation (PNF) and showed its efficacy [16, 17]. However, these studies involved cases with mild motor paralysis and movable joints. In contrast, PNF has not been shown to be effective for severely plegic hands without finger extension.

The facilitation conditions used in the current study differ from those in PNF. Thus, the method presented here is a new type of facilitation, although the conditions of "resistance exercise of the fixed joints" and "application of pressure on the joints" are similar to 2 of the 11 facilitation conditions defined by Kabat [16]. In manual facilitation, contraction of the extensor digitorum muscle does not occur, and facilitation fails if an interphalangeal joint is bent. In the method used in this study, the wrist, interphalangeal, and other joints must be fixed, but many joints in the hand are flexible, which makes complete manual fixation difficult. Moreover, passive joint compression transiently excites spinal motor nerve cells [18], which suggests that the facilitation effect of the extensor digitorum muscle will not occur without application of homogenous pressure to all the interphalangeal joints. Therefore, a thermoplastic splint that fitted the hyperextended plegic hand fingers was made for each subject. This custom-made splint was important for ensuring that the facilitation effect was obtained. The site and resistance to be applied during pushing of the plegic hand have to be determined by the therapist beforehand, and each subject may need a specific setting. Therefore, the UR-System-PARKO may be an appropriate robotic device for facilitating training of the extensor digitorum muscle in a manner that cannot be achieved by simple rehabilitation training. Further accumulation of data is required to evaluate the efficacy of the UR-System-PARKO.

## Acknowledgements

We are grateful to all the therapists, physicians, and trainers that participated in subject recruitment, evaluation, and training. A special thanks to Professor Takahiko Turumi for his guidance and participation. The authors also thank Dr. Toru Nagao for her consultation and assistance with the statistical methodology. This work was supported by JSPS KAKENHI Grant Number JP16K01544.

## Author details

Hirofumi Tanabe[1]*, Munehiro Ikuta[1], Toshimasa Mikawa[1], Akihiko Kondo[2] and Yoshifumi Morita[3]

1 Shonan Medical Sciences, Japan

2 Aso Rehabilitation College, Japan

3 Nagoya Institute of Technology, Japan

*Address all correspondence to: hirofumi.tanabe@sums.ac.jp

## References

[1] Steven W, Olf C, Carolee J, Winstein F, Miller JP, Paul A, et al. The EXCITE trial: Retention of improved upper extremity function among stroke survivors receiving CI movement therapy. The Lancet Neurology. Jan 2008;**7**(1):33-40

[2] Whitall J, McCombe WS, Silver K, Macko R. Repetitive bilateral arm training with rhythmic auditory cueing improves motor function in chronic hemiparetic stroke. Stroke. 2007;**38**(5):2390-2395

[3] Bonifer N, Anderson K. Application of constraint-induced movement therapy for an individual with severe chronic upper-extremity hemiplegia. Physical Therapy. 2003;**83**(4):384-398

[4] Bonifer N. Constraint-induced movement therapy after stroke: Efficacy for patients with minimal upper-extremity motor ability. Archives of Physical Medicine and Rehabilitation. 2005;**86**:1867-1873

[5] Nakayama H et al. Recovery of upper extremity function in stroke patients: The Copenhagen stroke study. Archives of Physical Medicine and Rehabilitation. 1994;**75**:394-398

[6] Kabat H. Studies on neuromuscular dysfunction. The role of central facilitation restoration of motor function in paralysis. Archives of Physical Medicine. 1952;**33**:521-533

[7] Chae J et al. Neuromuscular stimulation for upper extremity motor and functional recovery in acute hemiplegia. Stroke. 1998;**29**:975-979

[8] Yau Wang R. Effect of proprioceptive neuromuscular facilitation on the gait of patients with hemiplegia of long and short duration. Physical Therapy. 1994;**74**:1108-1115

[9] Tanabe H, Nagao T, Tanemura R. Application of constraint-induced movement therapy for people with severe chronic plegic hand. Asian Journal of Occupational Therapy. 2011:7-14

[10] Tanabe H. The Approach That Recovers for a Central Nerve Disorder-TANABE Therapy. Human Press; 2016

[11] Tanabe H, Mitsukane M, Toya N, Takeichi R, Hattori H, Morita Y, et al. Clinical evaluation of UR-system 2 for recovery of motor function of plegic upper limb after stroke. Journal of Robotics, Networking and Artificial Life. 2016;**3**(1):33-36

[12] Smith A. The coactivation of antagonist muscles. Canadian Journal of Physiology and Pharmacology. 1981;**59**:733-747

[13] Hogan N. Adaptive control of mechanical impedance by coactivation of antagonist muscles. IEEE Transactions on Automatic Control. 1984;**29**(8):681-690

[14] Morita Y, Toya N, Takeichi R, Hattori H, Tanabe H, Takagi Y, et al. Development of 'UR-system 2′: A training system for recovery of motor function of plegic upper limb after stroke. Advanced Robotics. 2016;**30**(21):11. ISSN:0169-1864 (Print)

[15] Tanabe H, Mitsukane M, Toya N, Takeichi R, Hattori H, Morita Y, Takagi Y, Hasegawa N. Clinical evaluation of UR-System 2 for recovery of motor function of plegic upper limb after stroke. Journal of Robotics, Networking and Artificial Life. June 2016;**3**(1):33-36

[16] Ray YW. Effect of proprioceptive neuromuscular facilitation on the gait

of patients with hemiplegia of long and short duration. Physical Therapy. 1994;**19**:1008-1115

[17] Dickstein R, Hocherman S, Pillar T, Shaham R. Stroke rehabilitation. Three exercise therapy approaches. The Physical Therapy. 1986;**66**(8):1233-1238

[18] Yanagisawa K, Fujiwara T, Takagi A. Effects of join tap proximation for lower extremities in normal adult subjects and hemiplegic patients. In: 10th International Congress of the WCPT, Proceedings; 1964. pp. 590-593

Chapter 4

# An Active Exoskeleton Called P.I.G.R.O. Designed for Unloaded Robotic Neurorehabilitation Training

*Guido Belforte, Terenziano Raparelli, Gabriella Eula, Silvia Sirolli, Silvia Appendino, Giuliano Carlo Geminiani, Elisabetta Geda, Marina Zettin, Roberta Virgilio and Katiuscia Sacco*

## Abstract

The development of innovative robotic devices allows the design of exoskeletons for robotic neurorehabilitation training. This paper presents the active exoskeleton called pneumatic interactive gait rehabilitation orthosis (P.I.G.R.O.), developed by the authors. The main innovative characteristic of this prototype is its design for fully unloaded robotic neurorehabilitation training, specific for brain-injured patients. It has six degrees of freedom (DOF) in the sagittal plane, an active ankle joint (removable if it is required); a wide range of anthropometric regulations, both for men and for women; a useful human machine interface (HMI); and an innovative harness system for the patient for the unloaded training. It is realized using light and strong materials, and it is electropneumatically controlled. In particular the authors also studied and defined some innovative input control curves useful for the unloaded training. In this paper, the main characteristics and innovations of P.I.G.R.O. are presented.

**Keywords:** active exoskeletons for unloaded robotic neurorehabilitation training, exoskeletons electropneumatic controlled, pneumatic actuators, robotic rehabilitation, lower limb exoskeletons

## 1. Introduction

Numerous studies in motor learning and neurorehabilitation training use robots to guide the patient in specific movements, while the clinicians analyze the behavior of the human motor control using the results obtained.

In general, the robotic exoskeletons for rehabilitation can be passive devices or active devices, where electric or pneumatic motors are used on the human upper or lower limb joints [1–10].

The use of robotic devices improves the neurorehabilitation trainings, their duration, and number [1, 2]. Many of these devices, used for rehabilitation on lower limbs, work with a fixed station and use a treadmill; generally they have motors on the hip and knee joints [8, 9], while the ankle joint is free. In fact in the traditional neurorehabilitation training, the patient walks on a treadmill, and he is connected to a harness and counterweights to reduce the body weight [8].

Nowadays a rehabilitation robot simulates the pattern of the normal walking gait and leads the movement of each lower limb. It can also correct the gait pattern of hemiplegic patients, collecting all the data [9, 10]. In the robotic devices, the use of a treadmill allows repetitive and specific movements to be carried out, which can improve the work of the muscles and the coordination of the movement in the patients [1].

The advantage of using an active exoskeleton without a fixed station is the possibility for the patient to move into the room, walking partially unloaded and helping by means of a body weight support. In this way, the proper perception of the space and the equilibrium of the patient can be analyzed and improved.

Otherwise a treatment with the patient completely unloaded avoids the activation of the antigravity musculature, and the effects of underwater treatments can be simulated.

Furthermore an unloaded training allows to increase, if it is necessary, some range of movement (ROM) of the joints, improving the stimulation of the motor cortex.

An unloaded training also allows to use different input control curves, if it is required by the clinicians, from the curves proper of the physiological gait cycle on the ground, carrying out special training studied for the patient's disease or useful for motor learning studies with healthy volunteers.

Often the unloaded trial is important in the beginning of the neurorehabilitation training for starting the rehabilitation work with the patient [11, 12].

From the robotic and the bioengineering experience, developed in the Department of Mechanical and Aerospace Engineering (DIMEAS) of Politecnico di Torino (Italy), an innovative active exoskeleton for unloaded robotic neurorehabilitation training was developed by the authors. It is called pneumatic interactive gait rehabilitation orthosis (P.I.G.R.O.) [11–18]. It is called Pneumatic Interactive Gait Rehabilitation Orthosis (P.I.G.R.O.) [11–18] and its design is developed through the continuous co-operation of engineers and doctors, allowing the realization of a final prototype that was patented by the Politecnico di Torino [14]. Afterward a spin-off for an industrial process design of the prototype was established in May 2017. In June 2015, P.I.G.R.O. was selected as one of the five more interesting projects in the Soft Landing program, APAC Innovation Summit 2015 Series—Robotics—Hong Kong, June 22–27, 2015. Furthermore, in June 2017, during the 26th International Conference on Robotics in Alpe-Adria-Danube Region, RAAD2017, P.I.G.R.O. authors received the Gold Best Application Paper Award [18].

In this paper, the exoskeleton P.I.G.R.O. is presented, useful for completely unloaded training with adult patients (both women and men).

## 2. Materials and methods

Comparing P.I.G.R.O. with other exoskeletons [19–22], it is possible to underline the following considerations.

In [19] an innovative assistive rehabilitation strategy is proposed by means of a wearable exoskeleton used without a treadmill and a body weight support. Here the dynamic stability of the patient is obtained by means of an efficient real-time stiffness adaptation for multiple joints (adaptive control system for assistive walking). In [20] an innovative robotic exoskeleton, designed as an ambulatory device, is presented and used during gait trainings on the ground. An adaptive strategy control is developed to guide the patient's legs in a specific gait pattern. In [21] an adaptive control model, controlled by means of the user intention, is proposed using an

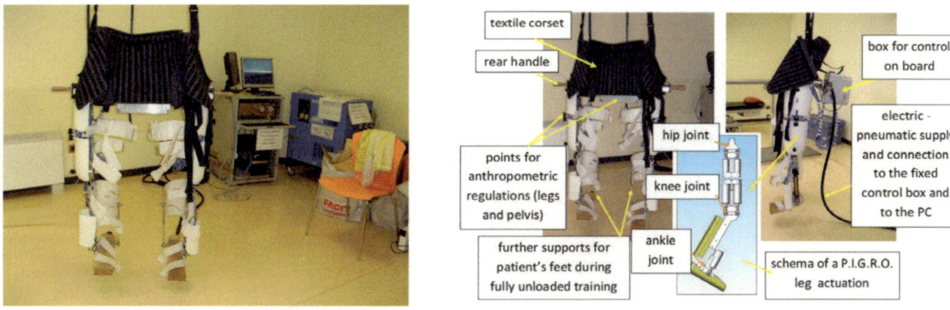


(a) (b)

**Figure 1.**
*(a) P.I.G.R.O. structure and (b) some P.I.G.R.O. details.*

exoskeleton for lower limb. The study is particularly referred to spinal cord-injured patients. The aim of this assistive control device is the user gait initiation and assistance in real time. This system was tested using a wearable exoskeleton: this shows the reliability of the control equipment in order to ensure the dynamic stability of the user. In [22] an interesting review about hybrid exoskeletons use to restore the gait cycle after a spinal cord injury is presented.

In comparison with the other exoskeletons, P.I.G.R.O. shows some different characteristics, as it was designed for fully unloaded training.

In **Figure 1** some details of P.I.G.R.O. are shown.

An unloaded treatment is useful in the beginning of the neurorehabilitation program especially for brain-injured patients [12].

Through several experimental tests, the authors also studied and defined some specific control input curves in the system suitable for the unloaded training [17].

In particular P.I.G.R.O. is not a device for walking assistance. It is an active exoskeleton designed for robotic neurorehabilitation purpose, and it can be only used in specific rehabilitation centers by clinicians and never with the patient alone. Its main field of application is training for patient with brain lesions affecting motor circuits.

### 2.1 The structure and the main characteristics of P.I.G.R.O.

The authors analyzed several aspects during the design of this active exoskeleton for unloaded neurorehabilitation training, such as the kinds of trainings to do with the device; the possibility to work without a fixed station; a structure that is light, comfortable, flexible, easy, and quick to wear, and safe, with proper and wide anthropometric regulations, with a mass of about 30 kg; a proper and safe range of movement for each joint; an increased ROM in the ankle joint (possible if the patient is fully unloaded) useful for the motor cortex stimulation but removable if it is necessary; some flexibility of the structure in the frontal plane, in order to avoid a hard robotic gait cycle and to allow some movements of the patient's pelvis and legs also in the frontal plane; the kind of actuation; the values of the torques in the joints lower than those required in the physiological walking on the ground; the control system (here an electropneumatic control system) with some input control curves studied by the authors for the unloaded training; a human machine interface (HMI); a harness system to unload the patient; and an interface between the machine and the patient [12, 17].

All of these aspects were analyzed and solved, giving to P.I.G.R.O. own and useful characteristics.

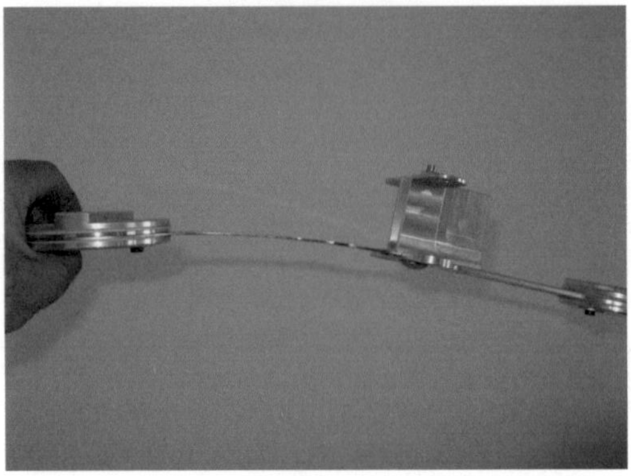

**Figure 2.**
*A detail of the P.I.G.R.O. leg flexibility.*

In particular P.I.G.R.O. includes the active exoskeleton (six DOF—degrees of freedom—in the sagittal plane with some possible little movements in the frontal plane too), moved using pneumatic cylinders and electropneumatic valves; a 10-m-long cable, in which both the tubes for the compressed air and the electric wires for the other source are collocated; a fixed box, where the final part of the electropneumatic control is located; a PC and two monitors, one for the operator and the other for the patient's biofeedback; and a movable compressor.

In order to allow some little movements of the patient's pelvis in the frontal plane too during the training, P.I.G.R.O. legs were built in C72 steel and in aluminum 7075 (Ergal) with a specific hardening treatment, giving to this exoskeleton a proper and useful flexibility.

**Figure 2** shows the possible deformation in a part of a P.I.G.R.O. leg.

The elements with movement (for the anthropometric regulation of femur and tibia length) have some Turcite© parts interposed in order to reduce the friction.

## 2.2 P.I.G.R.O. range of movement and anthropometric regulations

The range of movement in P.I.G.R.O. has 40° for the hip joint (from −20° to +20°), 60° for the knee joint (from 0° to 60°), and 40° for the ankle joint (from −25° to 15°). This last ROM is increased, in comparison with the range of the physiological walking on the ground, in order to improve the motor cortex stimulation during the unloaded training.

P.I.G.R.O. anthropometric regulations are between the 10%ile woman and 95%ile man [18], with a variation of the pelvis width from 300 mm, in the 10%ile woman, to 650 mm in the 95%ile man. The femur length varies from 370 mm, in the 10%ile woman, to 500 mm in the 95%ile man, and the tibia length varies from 360 mm, in the 10%ile woman, to 500 mm in the 95%ile man [23, 24]. These

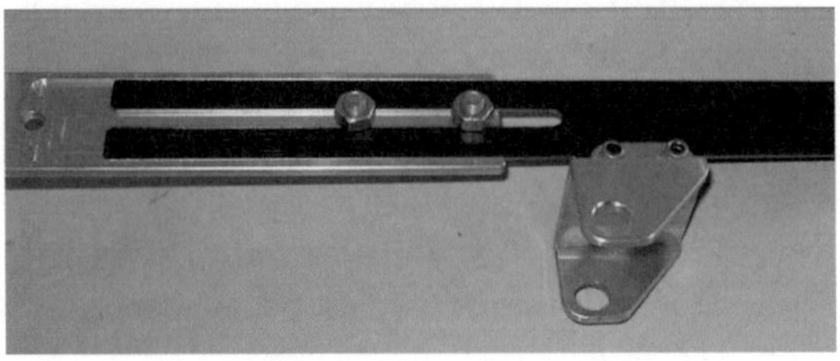

**Figure 3.**
*A detail of an anthropometric regulation in P.I.G.R.O.*

anthropometric regulations are done manually by the operator before the beginning of the trial. These regulations are obtained as the femur and the tibia of P.I.G.R.O. are both made of two rigid parts having a related movement, allowing the adjustment of the length required. Some Turcite© parts were interposed to reduce the friction. **Figure 3** shows a detail of an anthropometric regulation in P.I.G.R.O.

### 2.3 The pelvis regulation system design

On the back of the patient, P.I.G.R.O. has an adjustable structure, to which the two legs of the exoskeleton are connected, which allows the pelvis width to be regulated.

This structure has two screws, with one electric motor through which it is possible to increase or to decrease the pelvis width.

The movement can be conducted using a fast or a slow speed, selecting two different buttons. To this structure, the two legs of P.I.G.R.O. are connected, and two rigid bars, used also to guide the movement of the screws, are inside the structure and give it a strong rigid structure.

The geometry was obtained after several studies on various configurations, in order to design a system that allows a wide pelvis width regulation, that gives a proper speed during the pelvis width adjustment, that gives a strong support for P.I.G.R.O. legs, that provides two lateral supports through which the therapist can stabilize the patient's vertical position during the training, and that improves the wearability of P.I.G.R.O.

## 3. P.I.G.R.O. electropneumatic actuation design

In P.I.G.R.O. each joint is actuated by means of pneumatic cylinders.

In particular the choice of pneumatic actuators is due to the advantages existing in the compressed air, such as a soft and comfortable way of driving the patient's legs, an easy regulation of the forces during the training, and a safe and clean kind of actuation, useful for hospital applications.

**Figure 4** shows some details of the P.I.G.R.O. structure (**Figure 4a**) and of the P.I.G.R.O. activation design (**Figure 4b** and **c**).

**Figure 4b** shows a detail about the connection of the pneumatic cylinders in the hip and knee joints.

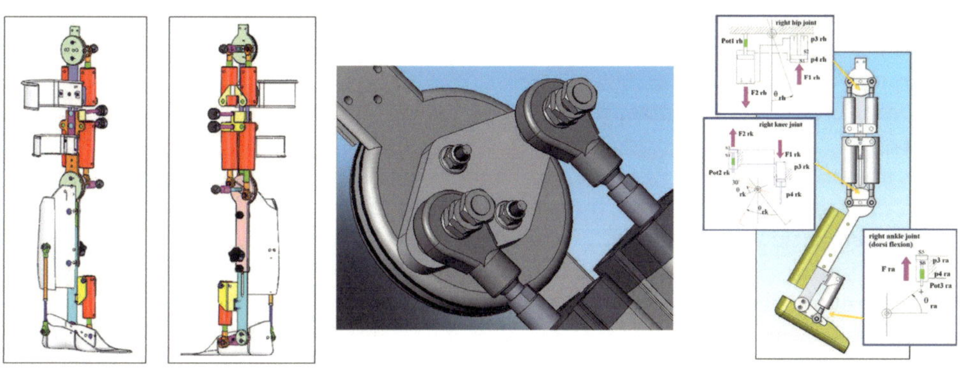


(a) (b) (c)

**Figure 4.**
*(a) P.I.G.R.O. complete structure, (b) a detail of the pneumatic cylinder connection, and (c) P.I.G.R.O. hip, knee, and ankle joints activation design.*

In **Figure 4c** the pneumatic activation of each joint of one leg of P.I.G.R.O. is shown. In particular an agonistic-antagonistic configuration, using cross-connected chambers, is used to connect the pneumatic cylinders of the hip and of knee joints.

This agonistic-antagonistic structure allows to have a proper surface for the actuator action, reduces the encumbrance of the system, if it is compared with the solution obtained with a single actuator in each joint, and gives a more equilibrated force in both directions of the movement of each cylinder. The ankle joint uses only one pneumatic actuator, when an unloaded training is carried out.

All of the movable elements are covered by means of proper protective caps for safety.

The pneumatic cylinders in P.I.G.R.O. are as follows: hip actuators bore 40 mm stroke 24 mm, knee actuators bore 40 mm stroke 35 mm, and ankle actuators bore 32 mm stroke 40 mm. With the maximum supply pressure ($6 \times 10^5$ Pa = 6 bar then used in the next text), the torque values for each joint are equal to hip joint, 45 Nm; knee joint, 45 Nm; and ankle joint, 25 Nm. These values are useful for the unloaded walking [17, 18].

In particular the evolution of the torque in each joint was evaluated versus the angle joint, observing a constant trend with a defined supply pressure.

Overall P.I.G.R.O. pneumatic actuation has also n.° 32 2/2 electropneumatic valves to control the cylinders. These valves are normally open and normally closed in order to realize a PID-PWM control system. The number of the electropneumatic valves was chosen in order to have a right conductance for the flow. Two electronic pressure regulators, put in the fixed box, allow the setting of the supply pressure value from the monitor of the operator.

Some more details on the electropneumatic circuit will be explained in the paragraph of the control system.

## 4. P.I.G.R.O. electropneumatic control system and the input control curves

The hardware of the control system has two main parts: a fixed control box with a PC, a keyboard, two monitors (one for the operator and the other for the patient's biofeedback), and a complementary equipment made of an onboard real-time control system with also the electropneumatic valves and the sensors.

In the fixed box, there is one card for the control and the data acquisition, as well as some electropneumatic valves for the P.I.G.R.O. pneumatic supply and emergency circuit. The onboard part has two cards, for the control and the data acquisition and for their transmission to the fixed box, the electropneumatic valves for the movement of the cylinders.

Some details of the electropneumatic control circuit of P.I.G.R.O. are shown in **Figure 5**.

As shown in **Figure 5**, P.I.G.R.O. has onboard n.° 10 pneumatic actuators; n.° 32 2/2 electropneumatic valves for the supply and for the vent of the actuators; n.° 12 pneumatic sensors, one for each cross-connected chamber of the actuators; and n.° 6 position sensors, one for each joint of each leg. The supply pressure in the actuators of the right and left legs can also be different during the test, and it can be increased or decreased, depending on what the training requires.

On the PC, a proper software for the control of the whole system and for the acquisition/analysis of the data is installed.

The realization and the configuration of the P.I.G.R.O. control system were carried out with the following steps.

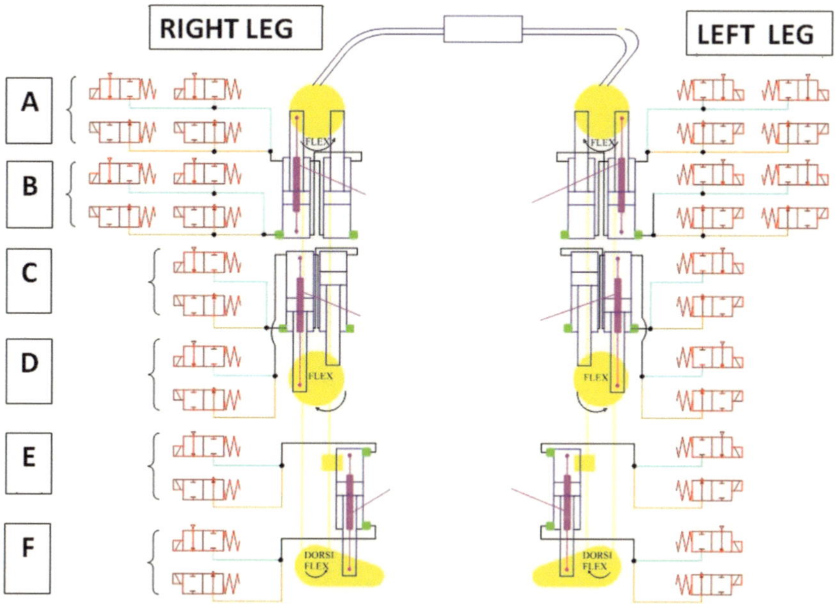


**Figure 5.**
*P.I.G.R.O. electropneumatic system onboard, with the electropneumatic valves and with the sensors. A = hip extension; B = hip flexion; C = knee flexion; D = knee extension; E = ankle plantarflexion; F = ankle dorsiflexion; in magenta = potentiometers; in green = pressure transducers.*

### 4.1 The definition of the reference system

In order to control properly the movement of each joint, a reference system for the P.I.G.R.O. legs joints is established, as shown in **Figure 6**. In particular, in **Figure 6** the reference system is referred to the right leg, seen in the sagittal plane from an external point of view. In P.I.G.R.O. it is possible to use various kinds of input control curves (required by the doctors) and, if it is necessary, different input control curves for the right and left leg.

### 4.2 The study and the definition of the input control curves useful for the unloaded training

The curves of a physiological gait cycle on the ground were analyzed and studied by the authors. As in this step, P.I.G.R.O. is designed for a completely unloaded training; several tests were carried out by the authors in order to define some input control curves suitable for this application [17].

In **Figure 7(a)** and **(b)**, the curves of the physiological walking on the ground (a) and the curves defined by the authors for the unloaded walking (b) are shown. In **Figure 7(a)** some red circles illustrate the main points of the difference between the physiological and the unloaded curves, such as the points where the contact between the foot and the ground occurs (points absent in the unloaded walking); the shape in some parts of the joints curves; the ROM of the ankle joint, increased for the unloaded walking; and some variations in the increasing/decreasing trend of the hip-knee-ankle angle joint curves [17].

The curves of **Figure 7(b)** reproduce the human gait cycle in a fully unloaded condition and allow a proper treatment of the patient during this rehabilitation step. Some experimental tests carried out controlling P.I.G.R.O. with these curves defined for the unloaded walking show their reliability.

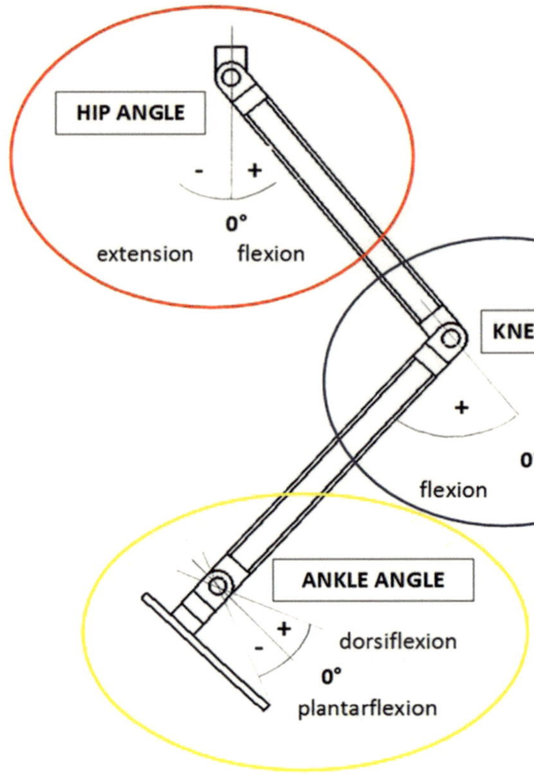


**Figure 6.**
*P.I.G.R.O. main reference system.*

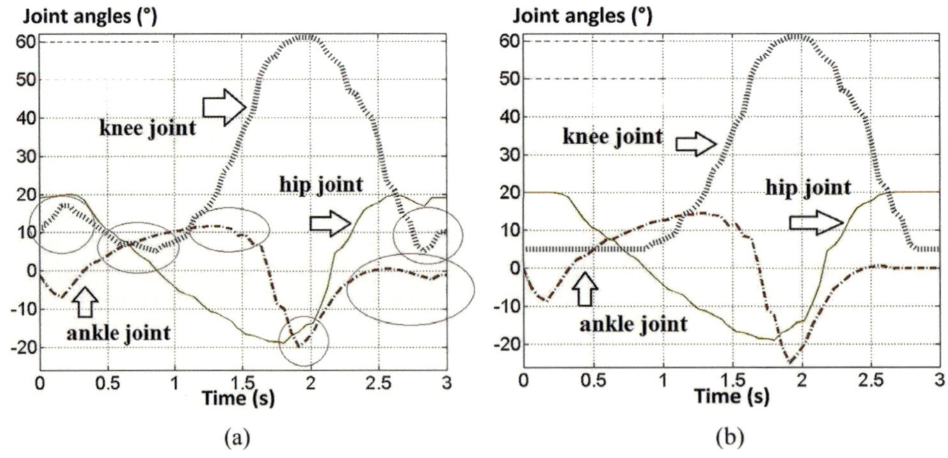


**Figure 7.**
*(a) Curves of the physiological walking on the ground and (b) authors' unloaded walking set curves (AUWS) [17].*

## 4.3 The definition of the structure of the P.I.G.R.O. control system for each joint

The control of P.I.G.R.O. is a real-time position control with a close loop for each joint, where a control subsystem was designed made of a PID-PWM control position structure, as shown in **Figure 8**.

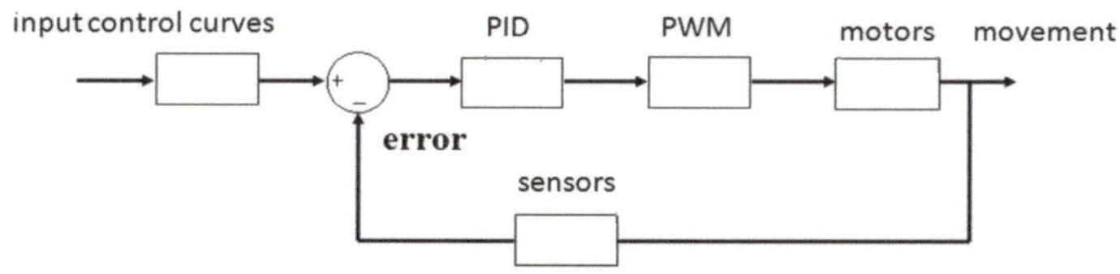


**Figure 8.**
*P.I.G.R.O. control structure for each lower limb joint.*

The input signal in each subsystem is the control curves selected and then compared with the position sensor signals (feedback) generating the "error."

The error is properly treated in order to control the electropneumatic valves.

The error sign establishes which types of electropneumatic valves (supply valves or discharge valves) have to be activated for the flexion or the extension of the joint.

The output signal of the PID controller is the input signal for the PWM part of the control system.

### 4.4 The definition of the parameters of the PWM and PID controller

The configuration of P.I.G.R.O. control system was carried out with a lot of experimental tests, done with a preliminary prototype of a single joint with two pneumatic actuators built with an agonistic-antagonistic structure, using cross-connected chambers and some masses to simulate the load.

Then other tests were done with a first prototype of P.I.G.R.O. made of a single leg, in particular the right leg, carrying out tests changing PWM carrier wave frequency, PID gains, tube diameters, and the number of the electropneumatic valves.

Finally the tests on the whole complete P.I.G.R.O. structure were carried out establishing the final configuration of the control system.

All of these tests allowed to establish the number of the electropneumatic valves (**Figure 5**) useful for a right control of the actuators, the tube diameters, and the parameters of the PID-PWM controller.

In particular the PWM characteristics were defined by varying the PWM carrier wave frequency and looking for its optimum values (**Figure 9a** and **b**).

The study was carried out using the exoskeleton with some healthy subjects, analyzing the effect of the carrier wave frequency values on the hip-knee-ankle

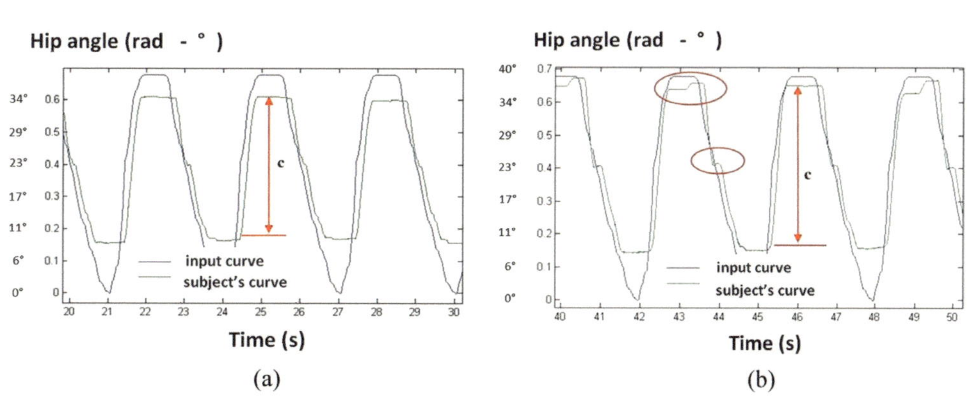


**Figure 9.**
*Tests on the hip joint, varying the PWM carrier wave frequency (female subject with a body mass of 58 kg; supply pressure, 6 bar; (a) PWM carrier wave frequency = 10 Hz and (b) PWM carrier wave frequency = 50 Hz).*

joint curves versus time, in comparison with the input trajectories. In this way, the optimum value for this frequency was defined.

In this step, the PID controller gains were not varied. As can be seen in **Figure 9a**, for the hip joint, for example, a low carrier wave frequency limits the actuator strokes and causes some oscillations in the subject curve.

On the other hand, a too much high carrier wave frequency (**Figure 9b**) improves the movement of the cylinders, but the subject's curve becomes less stable, and the oscillations increase.

After several experimental tests with healthy female and male volunteers, the optimum values of the PWM carrier wave frequency were defined for the hip-knee-ankle joints, obtaining a proper and stable movement of the actuators [11].

Then, the optimum values for the PID controller gains were investigated, testing the exoskeleton with healthy male/female subjects, with different body masses [11].

The PID controller gains are obtained, analyzing the kp proportional component, the ki integrative component (here always equal to zero), and the kd derivative component. Often these gains have different numerical values for the various parts of the input joint curves (initial, middle, and final part [17]).

The tests carried out allow to define the numerical values for the PID controller gains, which are values for subjects with body mass from 50 to 70 kg and values for subjects with body mass from 70 to 100 kg. In the beginning of the training, these PID controller gains are automatically selected by the software, as in the input data of the software; the patient's body mass is always required before the start of the trial.

In particular in the PID controller, the optimum values of the various components are defined as follows.

#### *4.4.1 Proportional component (kp)*

This component gives more or less reaction in the response of the system, so the authors used this component with different values in the various parts of each joint input control curves (i.e., hip-knee-ankle joints). The value of kp is higher when the inclination of the curve is higher. In particular the meaning of the kp in the parts of the curves of each joint is hip joint (increasing part of the hip input control curve kp_Ah, decreasing part of the hip input control curve kp_Al, constant part of the hip input control curve kp_Avl), knee joint (increasing and decreasing part of the knee input control curve kp_Gh, constant part of the knee input control curve kp_Gl), and ankle joint (increasing part of the ankle input control curve kp_Cl; decreasing part of the ankle input control curve kp_Ch).

#### *4.4.2 Integrative component (ki)*

In this system ki is always equal to zero because it can produce a block of the joint due to a saturation condition in the control.

#### *4.4.3 Derivative component (kd)*

kd increases the speed of the response of the system, but it can produce some oscillations. The authors decided to use for it a constant value for each curve (kd_A for the hip curve, kg_G for the knee curve, kd_C for the ankle curve). This value was then increased slowly till reaching a proper functioning of the system.

**Figure 10** show the use of some PID controller components in the hip-knee-ankle joint curves.

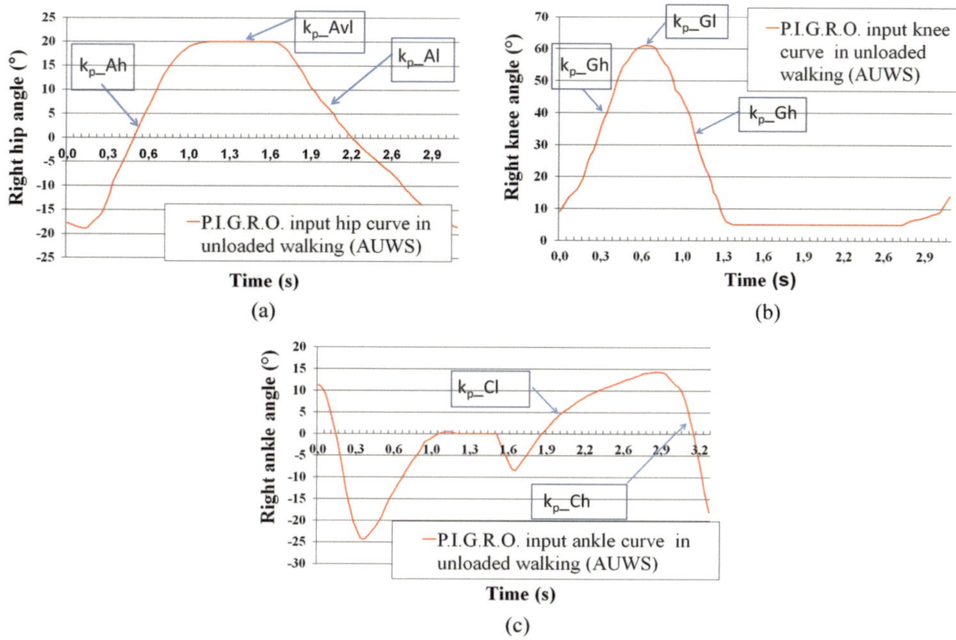


**Figure 10.**
*Details of some components of the PID controller referred to the hip (a) knee, (b) ankle, and (c) input control curves defined by the authors for the unloaded walking [17].*

## 5. The human machine interface of P.I.G.R.O.

P.I.G.R.O. has a useful human machine interface, which was properly developed. In particular there are two monitors, one for the operator and the other one for the patient's biofeedback.

In the human machine interface of P.I.G.R.O., it is possible to create and to save a file for each patient with all the patient's parameters; to start or to stop the system at the end of the training or during the training, if it is necessary; to change the input control curves, selecting them from a database created under the Doctors requirements; to show and to save the graphs obtained; to change the pressure in each leg, in the beginning of the training or during it; to save the time when this variation is done; and to have a proper biofeedback for the patient.

In particular, in the monitor for the operator (**Figure 11**), the behavior of the three joints of each leg (hip, knee, and ankle joint) can be analyzed during the trial by the clinicians. The graphs on the operator monitor can be saved.

In the panel of the operator, there are various buttons used to regulate the pressure in each leg independently and to stop the system at the end of the training, during the training, or in a possible emergency situation.

The supply pressure can be changed and its value in the two legs of P.I.G.R.O. can be different or equal, as the doctors require.

In fact a different value of pressure in the two legs of P.I.G.R.O. can be useful when the patient's pathology gives an asymmetric condition between the right and the left part of his body.

The time when the supply pressure is changed during the training can be saved.

Through the monitor for the operator, the duration of the whole training or of one part of the training can be registered and saved. In the program elaborated for P.I.G.R.O., there is the possibility to stop the patient's leg movement during the

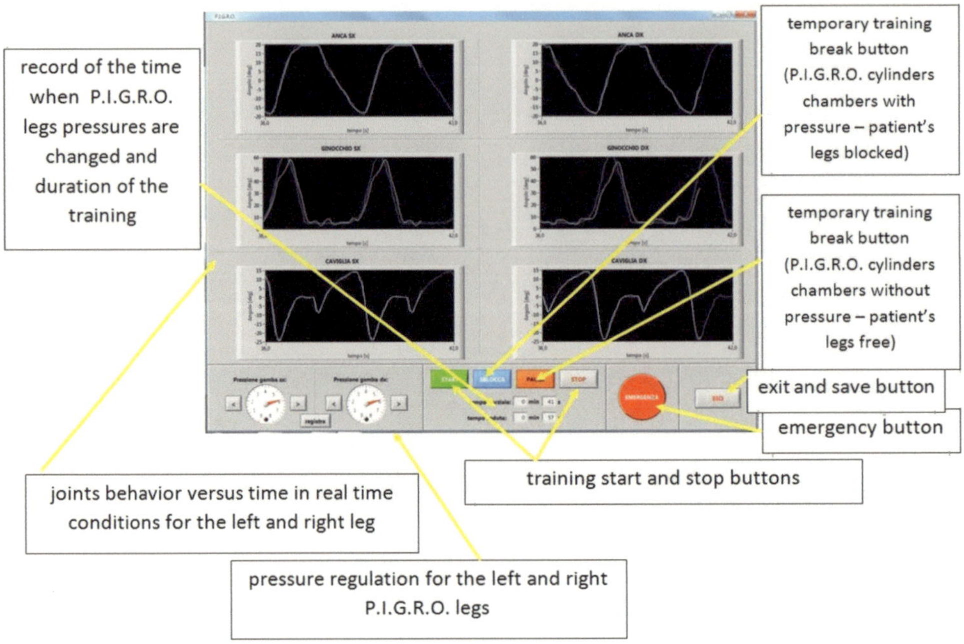


**Figure 11.**
*Some details of the HMI of P.I.G.R.O.*

training, closing the vent valves ports of all the actuators and having a pressure level in all the chambers of the actuators.

The possibility to stop the patient's legs in a specific position is useful for the doctors to investigate the cognitive status of the patient, for example, asking him the position of one or both of the stopped legs.

The patient's biofeedback has a monitor and the possibility of selecting one joint for one leg or the same two joints of the two legs.

In particular the biofeedback monitor shows, for each joint, that the patient's curve is within a certain range, if he is performing well.

P.I.G.R.O. has three emergency buttons: one on the monitor (for the operator), one on the fixed box (for the operator), and one to put in the hand of the patient.

During an emergency situation, all the electropneumatic valves of P.I.G.R.O. are switched to a vent configuration, with the possibility to immediately discharge all of the chambers of the actuators.

In this way, the patient can move autonomously his legs, while the training is immediately stopped.

Furthermore, the program allows to save all the data in files capable of being elaborated using many types of software.

## 6. The harness system for the patient and the textile corset of P.I.G.R.O.

As in this step of the research, P.I.G.R.O. is designed and used in unloaded training; a comfortable harness system for the patient was studied by the authors.

In fact, during the unloaded training, the patient is suspended by means of a harness system connected to the body weight support.

The exoskeleton P.I.G.R.O. is also connected to the body weight support by means of some proper belts and wore by the patient.

**Figure 12** shows the harness system for the unloaded training.

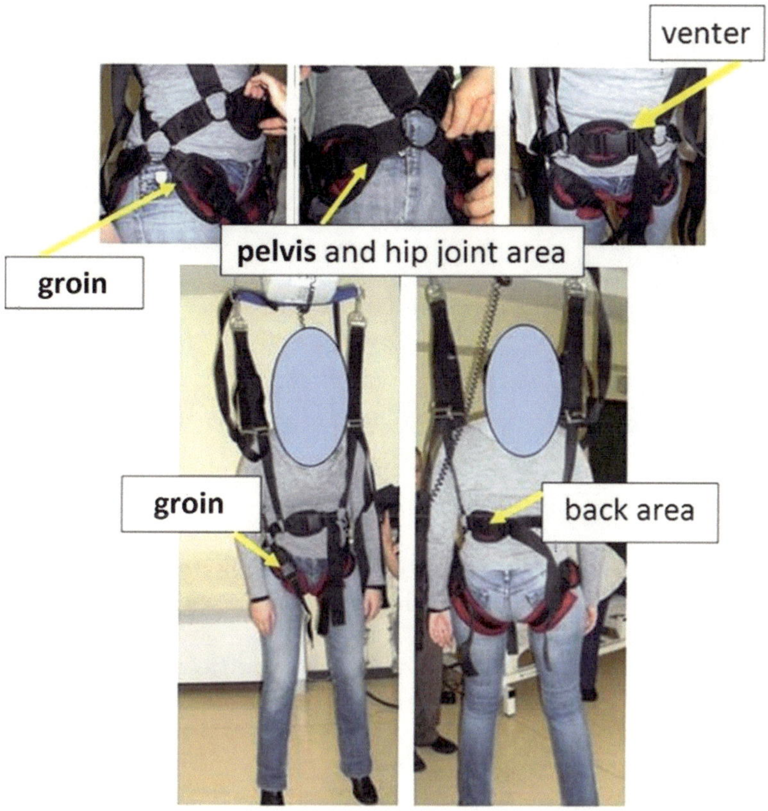


**Figure 12.**
*P.I.G.R.O. patient harness system for unloaded training.*

P.I.G.R.O. harness system supports a wide range of regulations and two specific configurations, one for men and the other for women.

This system was obtained after several studies on suspended people devices, in order to define the best design for the unloaded training done with P.I.G.R.O.

Its main characteristics are very comfortable and easy to wear; capable of suspending the patient in a vertical position, with the legs vertically extended; a proper and wide possibility of movement of the patient's legs during the unloaded training; and a construction made with safe and washable materials.

This harness system is partly made of textile parts, which are connected together by means of rigid rings, and some elements, filled of soft material, were also designed to improve the contact between the patient and the harness system and to avoid any pain for him.

In particular to define the best geometry of this harness system, a lot of considerations were done on the harness configuration in the hip joint area (**Figure 12**), where some differences from woman to man have to be foreseen, and the harness configuration on the patient's venter-groin-back area in order to obtain a very comfortable and safe design.

The purpose of this device is to sustain the patient in a vertical position for a trail duration of about 1 h, without any pain perception, which can reduce the benefit of the treatment and can cause irregularity in the movement during the trial.

A textile corset (**Figure 13**) was also studied to connect P.I.G.R.O. to the chest of the patient.

The choice of textile structures gives wear ability and comfort to the system, as these materials allow to adapt the device easily to men and to women from 10%ile

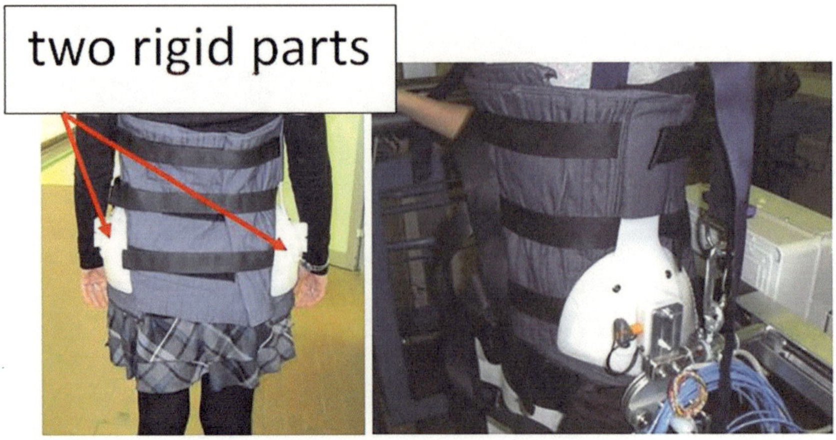


**Figure 13.**
*Textile corset, used to connect the patient to P.I.G.R.O.*

Italian woman to 95% Italian man. Furthermore a textile structure is safe and comfortable for the patient, as it avoids him any contact with rigid parts during the rehabilitation training.

This textile corset is somewhat regulated using an efficient system of straps sewed on the textile surface. The system makes it very wearable for patients with different body shapes.

In **Figure 13** some details were shown. Two lateral rigid elements, inserted in the external part of the textile corset, allow to connect it to the P.I.G.R.O. structure.

These two rigid parts can be connected or disconnected to P.I.G.R.O. legs by means of a proper lock device that allows a very quick and safe connection/disconnection, also if an emergency situation occurs.

## 7. Procedure defined to wear P.I.G.R.O. on the patient

The authors also defined a proper procedure to wear P.I.G.R.O. on the patient, verifying the wear ability and the comfort of the system and the possibility to wear P.I.G.R.O. on the patient in a short time.

The main steps of this procedure are measure on the distances between hip-knee and knee-ankle of the patient and the pelvic width in order to do the anthropometric regulations in the P.I.G.R.O. structure; insert these measures in the P.I.G.R.O. software, together with the patient's weight and the patient's data; wear the harness system on the patient; wear P.I.G.R.O. on the patient; verify all the system; and then unload the patient and P.I.G.R.O. using the body weight support.

In **Figure 14** a detail for the right use of the patient's harness system is shown: the unloaded walking training requires a proper vertical position of the patient.

In particular P.I.G.R.O. ankle joint has also a proper support for the patient's foot.

To guarantee that the patient's foot remains in a horizontal plane, the authors designed two screws, put in the inside part of the two P.I.G.R.O. legs, connected between the tibia blade and the foot support.

The regulation of these screws allow to have a right posture of the patient's feet during the unloaded walking cycle.

In **Figure 15** some details of this system and of its regulation were shown.

The average time to wear P.I.G.R.O. on a patient is about 20 min.

As the study is still in progress, the authors do not explain in this phase of the research more details on the tests carried out and the results obtained.

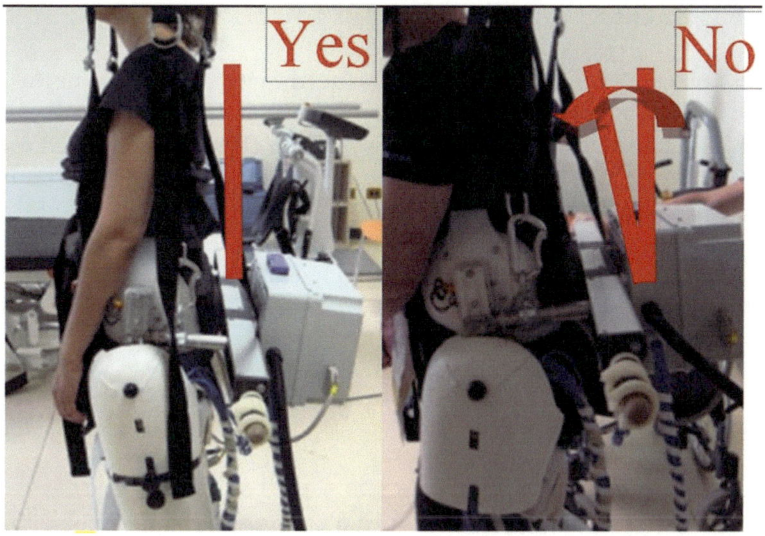


**Figure 14.**
*Some details of the right position of the suspended patient for the unloaded training.*

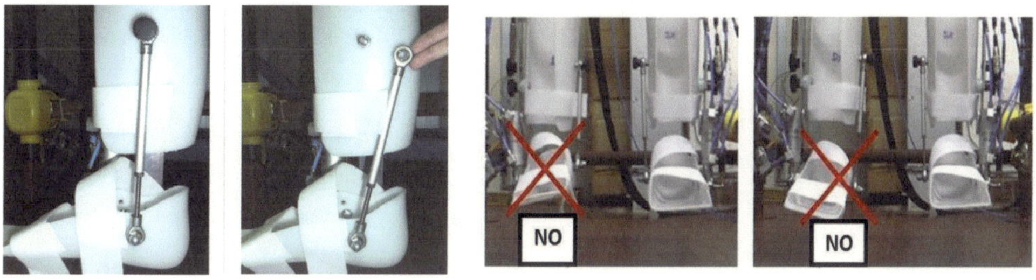


**Figure 15.**
*(a) Screw inside each leg of P.I.G.R.O. to support the rigid part for the patient foot and (b) some details of regulation of this screw.*

## 8. Conclusions

This article illustrates the structure and the main and innovative characteristics of P.I.G.R.O., an active electropneumatically controlled exoskeleton for unloaded robotic neurorehabilitation training. It is constructed to work without a fixed station, as this procedure is useful in the beginning of the trial to avoid the activation of the antigravity musculature.

P.I.G.R.O. has a real-time position control.

A useful human machine interface was developed: it allows P.I.G.R.O. to be easily used. It is possible to insert, to acquire, to save the patient's data, to carry out properly and safely various kinds of training, and to analyze the data. An innovative, useful, and comfortable harness system for the patients' unloaded training was studied and developed.

The preliminary tests show the reliability and the importance of this active exoskeleton that is also easy to wear.

In the future, the study of P.I.G.R.O. used in a walking training on the ground will be carried out, and some more experimental tests will be conducted in order to understand other possible improvements of this exoskeleton.

## Acknowledgements

The work presented in this paper was financed, with funding from the Compagnia di San Paolo project, "Active exoskeleton for the functional gait rehabilitation of paretic patients," and with funding from the Piedmont regional administration project, entitled "Validation of a method for gait rehabilitation for paretic patients using an active orthosis" (2006–2008).

## Conflicts of interest

The Authors declare no conflict of interest.

## Thanks

Authors would like to thank the Puzzle Rehabilitation Center, Turin (Italy), for providing brain injury information, and Engrs. P. Bois, G. Castorina, A. Genta, Y. Han, G. Perricelli, F. Racca, and G. Viano for their help during this study.

## Author details

Guido Belforte[1,2], Terenziano Raparelli[3], Gabriella Eula[3*], Silvia Sirolli[2], Silvia Appendino[4], Giuliano Carlo Geminiani[5,6], Elisabetta Geda[7], Marina Zettin[8,9], Roberta Virgilio[8] and Katiuscia Sacco[5,6]

1 Former of Department of Mechanical and Aerospace Engineering, Politecnico di Torino, Torino, Italy

2 "NIMBLE ROBOTICS"—Spin Off of Politecnico di Torino, Torino, Italy

3 Department of Mechanical and Aerospace Engineering, Politecnico di Torino, Torino, Italy

4 Department of Applied Science and Technology, Politecnico di Torino, Torino, Italy

5 Imaging and Plasticity Research Group at Department of Psychology, University of Turin, Torino, Italy

6 Neuroscience Institute of Turin, Torino, Italy

7 Istituto Delle Riabilitazioni Riba-IRR, Torino, Italy

8 Puzzle Rehabilitation Center for Brain Injury, Torino, Italy

9 Department of Psychology, University of Turin, Torino, Italy

*Address all correspondence to: gabriella.eula@polito.it

## References

[1] Riener R, Lunenburger L, Colombo G. Human-centered robotics applied to gait training and assessment. Journal of Rehabilitation Research and Development. 2006;**43**:679-694. DOI: 10.1682/JRRD.2005.02.0046

[2] Wolbrecht ET, Chan V, Reinkensmeyer DJ, Bobrow JE. Optimizing compliant, model-base robotic assistance to promote neurorehabilitation. IEEE Transactions on Neural Systems and Rehabilitation Engineering. 2008;**16**:286-297. DOI: 10.1109/tnsre.2008.918389

[3] Huang VS, Krakauer JW. Robotic neurorehabilitation: A computational motor learning perspective. Journal of Neuroengineering and Rehabilitation. 2009;**6**:1-13. DOI: 10.1186/1743-0003-6-5

[4] Roy A, Krebs HI, Williams DJ, Bever CT, Forrester LW, Macko RM, et al. Robot-aided neurorehabilitation: A novel robot for ankle rehabilitation. IEEE Transactions on Robotics. 2009;**25**:569-582. DOI: 10.1109/TRO.2009.2019783

[5] Baker R. Gait analysis methods in rehabilitation. Journal of Neuroengineering and Rehabilitation. 2006;**3**:1-10. DOI: 10.1186/1743-0003-3-4

[6] Reinkensmeyer J, Dietz V, editors. Neurorehabilitation Technology. 2nd ed. Springer; 2016. 929 p. DOI: 10.1007/978-3-319-28603-7

[7] Dollar AM, Herr H. Lower extremity exoskeletons and active orthoses: Challenges and state-of-the-art. IEEE Transactions on Robotics. 2008;**24**:144-158. DOI: 10.1109/TRO.2008.915453

[8] Jezernik S, Colombo G, Keller T, Frueh H, Morari M. Robotic orthosis Lokomat: A rehabilitation and research tool. International Neuromodulation Society. 2003;**6**:108-115. DOI: 10.1046/j.1525-1403.2003.03017.x

[9] Krebs HI, Volpe BT, Aisen ML, Hogan N. Robotic applications in neuromotor rehabilitation. Topics in Spinal Cord Injury Rehabilitation. 1999;**5**:50-63. DOI: 10.1017/S0263574702004587

[10] Muro-de-la-Herran A, Garcia-Zapirain B, Mendez-Zorrilla A. Gait analysis methods: An overview of wearable and non-wearable systems, highlighting clinical applications. Sensors. 2014;**14**:3362-3394. DOI: 10.3390/s140203362

[11] Belforte G, Eula G, Appendino S, Sirolli S. Pneumatic interactive gait rehabilitation orthosis: Design and preliminary testing. Proceedings of the Institution of Mechanical Engineers, Part H. 2011;**225**:158-169. DOI: 10.1243/09544119JEIM803

[12] Sacco K, Cauda F, Duca S, Belforte G, Eula G, Gastaldi L, et al. A combined robotic and cognitive training for locomotor rehabilitation: Evidences of cerebral functional reorganization in two chronic traumatic brain injured patients. Frontiers in Human Neuroscience. 2011;**5**:1-9. DOI: 10.3389/fnhum.2011.00146

[13] Geda E, D'agata F, Geminiani G, Cauda F, Duca S, Zettin M, et al. Motor attention in procedural learning: Behavioral and cerebral changes. In: AISC 2011, Proceedings of the 8th Congress "Tecnologia, Scienze Umane e Scienze Della Salute"; 26-28 May Riva del Garda, Italy. Associazione Italiana Scienze Cognitive; 2011. pp. 111-115

[14] Belforte G, Eula G, Appendino S, Geminiani GC, Zettin M. Active orthosis for the motion neurological rehabilitation of lower limbs, system

comprising such orthosis and process for operating such system. Patent EP 2 825 146 B1

[15] Belforte G, Eula G, Sirolli S, Bois P, Geda E, D'Agata F, et al. Bra.Di.P.O. and P.I.G.R.O.: Innovative devices for motor learning programs. Journal of Robotics. 2014;**2014**:1-12. DOI: 10.1155/2014/656029

[16] Belforte G, Eula G, Ivanov A, Raparelli T, Sirolli S, Geminiani GC, et al. Rehabilitation and pneumatics for smart quality of life (SQOL) at Politecnico di Torino. In: Wheelchair Design Workshop. Tokyo, Japan. 2013. pp. 1-10

[17] Belforte G, Eula G, Sirolli S, Appendino S, Geda E, Geminiani G, et al. Control curves for a new lower limbs robotic exoskeleton obtained from the study of joints angles during an unloaded human walking. International Journal of Mechanics and Control. 2017;**18**:3-14

[18] Sacco K, Belforte G, Eula G, Raparelli T, Sirolli S, Geda E, et al. An active exoskeleton for robotic neurorehabilitation training driven by an electro-pneumatic control. In: Proceedings of the 26th International Conference on Robotics in Alpe-Adria-Danube Region RAAD2017; 21-23 June 2017; Politecnico di Torino, Torino, Italy. Advances in Service and Industrial Robotics—Springer; 2017. pp. 1-8

[19] Rajasekaran V, Aranda J, Casals A. Adaptive walking assistance based on human-orthosis interaction. In: 2015 IEEE/RSJ International Conference on Intelligent Robots and Systems (IROS); 28 September – 2 October 2015; Hamburg, Germany. IEEE; 2015. pp. 6190-6195

[20] Bortole M, del-Ama A, Rocon E, Moreno JC, Brunetti F, Pons JL. A robotic exoskeleton for overground gait rehabilitation. In: Proceedings—IEEE International Conference on Robotics and Automation (ICRA); 6-10 May 2013; Karlsruhe, Germany. IEEE; 2013. pp. 3356-3361

[21] Rajasekaran V, Lopez-Larras E, Trincado-Alonso F, Aranda J, Montesano L, del-Ama AJ, et al. Volition-adaptive control for gait training using wearable exoskeleton: Preliminary tests with incomplete spinal cord injury individuals. Journal of Neuroengineering and Rehabilitation. 2018;**15**:1-15. DOI: 10.1186/s12984-017-0345-8.

[22] del-Ama AJ, Koutsou AD, Moreno JC, de-los-Reyes A, Gil-Agudo A, Pons JL. Review of hybrid exoskeletons to restore gait following spinal cord injury. (JRRD)—Journal of Rehabilitation Research and Development. 2012;**49**:497-514. DOI: 10.1682/JRRD.2011.03.0043

[23] UNI EN ISO 7250-1:2010: Basic human body measurements for technological design—Part 1: Body measurement definitions and landmarks

[24] UNI EN ISO/TR 7250-2:2011: Basic human body measurements for technological design—Part 2: Statistical summaries of body measurements from individual ISO populations

## Section 4

# Surgical Planning

Chapter 5

# Surgical Planning and Additive Manufacturing of an Anatomical Model: A Case Study of a Spine Surgery

*Levent Aydin, Ozgur Cakir, Riza Dilek and Mucahit Ege*

## Abstract

3D scanning technologies have promising solutions for medical needs such as anatomical models, biocompatible implants, and orthotic/prosthetic models. Although virtual presurgical planning offers more precise results, it may not be applied in every hospital because of the high costs. The aim of this study is to assess the accuracy of the suggested low-cost and effective surgical planning method by means of additive manufacturing to increase success rate of each surgery. In this study, a full spine model of a scoliosis patient was acquired and reconstructed in MIMICS software using different filters and parameters. Therefore, a comparison in terms of geometrical errors among each model was performed based on a reference model. Subsequently, patient-specific full spine model was manufactured using a three-dimensional printing method (fused deposition modeling) and utilized before the surgery. 3D surgical model reconstruction parameters such as wrap tool, binomial blur, and curvature flow filters produced high geometrical errors, while mean filter produced the lowest geometrical error. Furthermore, similarity results of the curvature flow and discrete Gaussian filters were close to mean filter. Smooth tool and mean filter produced almost the same volume of the reference model. Consequently, an ideal protocol for surgical planning of a spine surgery is defined with measurable accuracy. Thus, success rate of a spine surgery may be increased especially for the severe cases owing to the more accurate preoperative review: operability.

**Keywords:** additive manufacturing, image guided surgery, orthopedic surgery, surgical planning, accuracy assessment, scoliosis

## 1. Introduction

Scoliosis is a three-dimensional (3D) deformity in the natural shape of spine that requires surgery in serious cases [1]. A lateral deviation of the spine greater than 10 degrees is accepted as scoliosis and an abnormal sideways curvature is observed from the frontal plane of a patient, while a healthy spine should look like straight [2, 3]. Although hereditary factors play a role in the etiology, most of the cases (80% of the patients) with unknown cause are called idiopathic scoliosis and classified into three main groups based on the age, namely, (i) infantile (up to 3 years old), (ii) juvenile (4–9 years old), and (iii) adolescent (10 years old to teen years) [4]. The severity of scoliosis is also determined by Cobb method that provides obtain information about the curvature of the spine in terms of degrees. According to these measurements, a scoliotic curve of the spine is defined as (i) mild scoliosis (10–25°, requires monitoring), (ii) significant scoliosis (25–40°, treated with bracing), and (iii) severe scoliosis (over 40°, requires surgery) [5]. Recently, a number of the scoliosis patients are growing up to 2–3% worldwide due to the unawareness of people [6]. It is important to predict risk of progression, diagnose at early stage for preventing degenerative effects, and contribute to the patient's quality of life. Unfortunately, in some cases, rapid progress on spine deformity or late diagnosis is resulted with surgical operations that are necessary to stabilize the spine by means of rod placement on each affected vertebra [6]. All operations require precise processes in a limited workspace because of the spinal nerves and blood vessels. Besides, an injury of a vessel around the surgical site may initiate clotting that may result with pulmonary embolism or even death [7]. Therefore, novel technologies and methods are of great importance to assist or plan the surgery in advance.

Medical imaging technologies such as multidetector computed tomography (MDCT) and magnetic resonance imaging (MRI) are rapidly evolving to visualize more complex tissues of the human body [8]. Furthermore, high-resolution images provide radiologists more accurate diagnosis [9]. Although 3D visualization of the scanned tissues simplifies the surgical procedures, patients may undergo a suboptimal outcome after the treatment [10]. On the other hand, two-dimensional (2D) computer screens prevent the direct interaction with the target 3D model [11]. While virtual presurgical planning offers more precise results and overcomes mentioned drawbacks above, it is not applicable for every hospital because of its high costs [10]. Additive manufacturing, layer-by-layer fabrication of a physical object, is increasingly being used especially in the fields of medicine. Nowadays, these technologies are utilized with medical imaging to produce patient-specific (i) medical devices, orthosis, and prosthesis [12], (ii) anatomical to assist-surgical models [13], (iii) body parts [14], (iv) dental and maxillofacial implants [15], (v) blood vessels [16], and (vi) organs [17]. Typical 2D digital imaging and communications in medicine (DICOM) files from the CT or MRI images are transformed into a 3D standard tessellation language (STL) file to perform 3D printing of the target model. A wide range of polymers including glass, ceramic, metal, or biological materials may be used to create complex models in a cost-effective way compared to conventional manufacturing methods [18]. Although the latest innovative studies are focused on a functional tissue or even an organ printing, clinical bedside applications of these technologies are difficult and limited [11]. On the other hand, surgical planning or patient-specific implant production via 3D printing is available for any case and widely used to manage a complex surgery or achieve the exact placement of an implant [18]. Consequently, success rate of each surgery is significantly increased as well as it becomes minimally invasive and requires shorter recovery owing to the preoperative review [19, 20].

Surgical planning by means of additive manufacturing consists of five basic steps, namely, (i) data acquisition, (ii) image segmentation, (iii) 3D model reconstruction, (iv) 3D printing, and (v) preoperative review [21]. In data acquisition step, a medical imaging system such as CT is used to obtain 2D DICOM images in general. The accuracy of surgical planning is first dependent on the contrast-to-noise ratio (CNR) of scanned raw images [22]. High CNR values provide detailed segmentation before the 3D reconstruction of a model. These images are then processed via a commercial (Materialize Mimics) or an open-source (InVesalius) medical image processing software using the default segmentation functions or manual selection of the region of interest on each image during the segmentation step. Thus, the target anatomical model's contour is masked on each image section. In 3D model reconstruction step, the mask images are positioned sequentially to form a solid model in 3D workspace of the software. Tissue-specific filters or data sets may be applied to minimize noise using predefined thresholds before and after the 3D reconstruction process. The solid model is exported as a STL file and prepared to be 3D printed. In 3D printing step, the STL file is 3D printed using one of the additive manufacturing methods such as fused deposition modeling (FDM), selective laser sintering (SLS), or stereolithography (SLA). In a preoperative review step, the printed model is evaluated and used before and during the surgery (requires sterilization) as a reference model that guide the operation as well as it can be used for custom implant or assistive surgical apparatus creation such as drill guides [23]. Since surgical planning is important and plays a crucial role during the surgery, reference 3D model requires to be created with minimal geometrical errors. The accuracy of 3D reconstructed models can be analyzed by calculating the Hausdorff distance (HD) and dice similarity coefficient (DSC) values for each model [24, 25]. While DSC measures the volume overlap between two models that ranges from 0 (no overlap) to 1 (exact overlap), HD calculates the Euclidean distance between each binary volume [26, 27]. Furthermore, several methods (geometric distance, roughness, structure, saliency, and strain-energy-based calculations) may be implemented to assess visual quality and accuracy of the 3D models [28]. In this study, a spine model of a scoliosis patient is first acquired and then 3D reconstructed in MIMICS software (manual and automatic segmentation) using different filters and parameters to compare each geometrical error. The results of the DSC and HD values of each reconstructed model reveal the ideal protocol for surgical planning of a spine surgery and determine the accuracy of the created model.

## 2. Material and methods

A 6-year-old patient (male) who has a congenital scoliosis history participated to this study for obtaining raw image data. Medical scanning process was performed at the Radiology Department, Faculty of Medicine Kocaeli University, using a CT scanner (Aquillion 64, Toshiba Medical Systems, Tokyo, Japan). Ethical permission was received by the Ethics and Research Committee of Kocaeli University (reference number, KU GOKAEK 2019/204). A full spinal CT scanning was performed at 2 mm of slice thickness, 140 mm field of view (FoV) and 135 kV (40 mA, 1 s). Raw DICOM images (449 slices) were obtained from the picture archiving and communication system (PACS) server of the Radiology Department (**Figure 1(a)**). Thus, data acquisition process, the first step of the surgical planning, was completed.

MIMICS software (v19) was utilized in image segmentation step, and a reference model was automatically reconstructed via MIMICS without any filters (**Figure 1(b)**). DICOM files (449 images) were imported, and segmentation process was performed using the thresholding tool at predefined threshold set of the bone (226, Hounsfield Unit, HU as lower threshold, and 3071 HU as higher threshold). These parameters were ideal to obtain exact contour of the target model in a maximum allowable noisy form according to the raw DICOM images for this case. Segmentation step was completed after each image section was masked and highlighted by a different color (**Figure 1(c)**).

3D calculation function was utilized at high quality to reconstruct the 3D raw surface, and a quite noisy model was created with desired contour based on the masked images in 3D model reconstruction step (**Figure 1(d)**). Each image

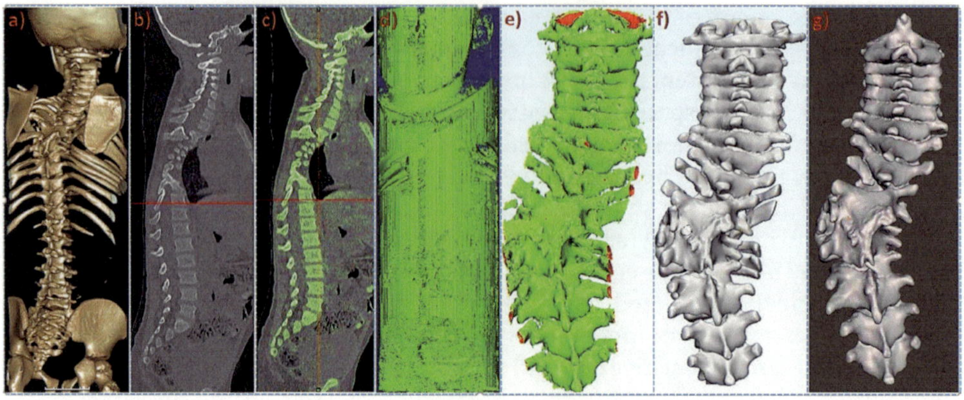


**Figure 1.**
*3D Surgical model segmentation of the reference model (a) An image of the 3D raw model, based on non-filtered DICOM images in Sectra workspace, a 3D DICOM viewer of the default system software that does not allow 3D model exporting or processing, (b) Importing non-filtered DICOM images in MIMICS, (c) Segmentation of each image and obtaining the exact contour of target model in a maximum allowable noisy form in MIMICS, (d) 3D reconstruction of the raw DICOM images in a noisy form via MIMICS, (e) Manual noise cleaning in 3-Matic, (f) Manual surface reconstruction and fixing the geometrical errors of 3D raw model in 3-Matic, (g) Fixing the sharp cornered bonded surfaces in Meshmixer.*

was positioned sequentially to form a 3D raw model of the spine. Since there was noise in the workspace and model's surface, the 3D raw model was directly exported to 3-matic software (v11, Materialize) for manual surface reconstruction and noise elimination (**Figure 1(e)**). The surface geometry of the model was manually revised, and the noise was manually cleared via 3-matic software according to the raw image geometries in MIMICS. Polygon area mark tool under the Mark—Area Mark menu was used to select each noisy surface and subsequently deleted. The gaps of the deleted surfaces were marked as bad contours on the 3D raw model. The bad contours were then selected and fixed, respectively, using the Fill Hole Freeform tool under the Fix menu. The Fill Hole Freeform process was performed at medium triangulation quality and created in tangent form. After manual surface reconstruction, the Fix Wizard tool under the Fix menu was utilized to fix geometrical normals, stitching, noise shells, holes, triangles, overlaps, and shells on the model. The errors were automatically fixed by clicking Follow Advice, Apply, and Update buttons, respectively, for each option (**Figure 1(f)**). Finally, the patient ID was added using the Quick Label tool under the Finish menu. Thus, 3D-reconstructed reference surgical model was obtained and exported as STL file by clicking File, Export, and STL buttons, respectively. The reference model was exported at binary format and one scaling factor. Some sharp cornered bonded surfaces that occurred by Fix Wizard tool during the fixing process were also revised in Meshmixer (v3.4.35, Autodesk) manually to obtain exact geometry of target anatomical model. Robust Smooth tool under the Sculp – Brushes menu was used (brush parameters, 10 strength, 10 size, 0 depth, and 0 laziness) to fix sharp surfaces (**Figure 1(g)**). The 3D model reconstruction step was completed after the reference model has taken its final shape (48 hours of work). 3D reconstruction of the reference surgical model is illustrated step by step in **Figure 1**.

Test models were separated into three groups, namely, (i) preprocessed, (ii) post-processed, and (iii) fully processed models. Preprocessed models were obtained using the filtered DICOM images before the segmentation step without any post-process in MIMICS. Post-processed models were created from the raw DICOM images and only processed via 3-matic after the model was

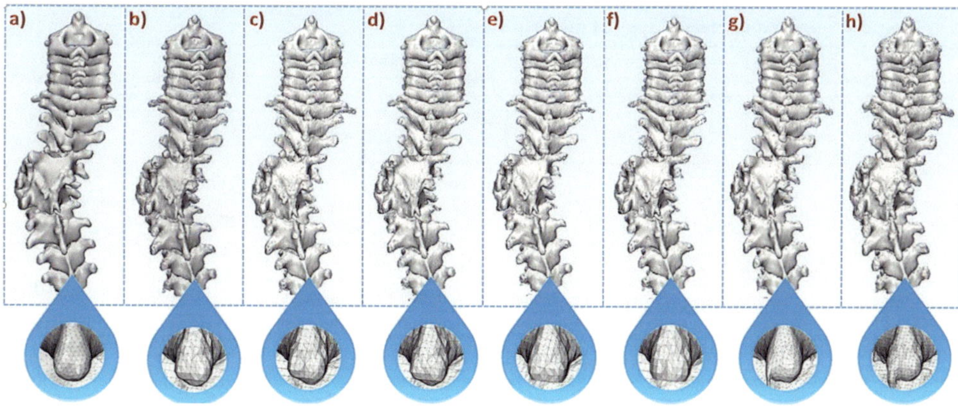


**Figure 2.**
*Reference model and each generated 3D test model with a local mesh view (a) Reference model, (b) Binomial blur filter in MIMICS, (c) Curvature flow filter in MIMICS, (d) Discrete gaussian filter in MIMICS, (e) Mean filter in MIMICS, (f) Median filter in MIMICS, (g) Smooth function in 3-Matic and (h) Wrap function in 3-Matic.*

reconstructed (**Figure 2(a)**). Fully processed models were formed with a combination of both processes. Five different image filters of MIMICS, (i) binomial blur (**Figure 2(b)**), (ii) curvature flow (**Figure 2(c)**), (iii) discrete Gaussian (**Figure 2(d)**), (iv) mean (**Figure 2(e)**), and (v) median (**Figure 2(f)**), were applied on the raw DICOM images, respectively, and then the segmentation step was performed separately for each sample on preprocessed models. Two different 3D tools of 3-matic, (i) Smooth (**Figure 2(g)**) and (ii) wrap (**Figure 2(h)**), were utilized separately for each sample in post-processing case. Preprocessing, post-processing, and full-processing parameters of the 3D reconstructed surgical models are given in **Table 1**.

Before the calculation of HD and DSC values by CloudCompare software, each spine model was processed via 3-matic software that was necessary to determine the spine regions equally on each sample model and obtain more correct results in accuracy assessment. Therefore, the spine sections of each model were extracted manually and exported using the default options. All test models were imported into the CloudCompare software (v2.11, Open Source) and then compared with the reference model in terms of the HD and DSC results [29]. The best results of the preprocessing and the post-processing cases were combined and applied together to form the fully processed model. Finally, the fully processed model was compared to the reference model to reveal the ideal solution for 3D surgical model reconstruction. Each generated test model is illustrated in **Figure 2**.

HD of the test models was calculated by means of importing and analyzing the 3D models, the reference model and one of the test models at the same time, in CloudCompare workspace. Both models were then aligned using Registration Match bounding function—under the Tools menu. This process is required to align the box centers (volume frames) of models before performing any similarity function in order to obtain accurate results. Fine registration function under the Tools—Registration menu was applied on each model to highlight the difference of point clouds without any scale adjustment. The fine registration function also applies a rotation to compared model (generates a rotation matrix with a theoretical overlap value) to provide an ideal Overlap in volumes of the both reference and compared test model. Finally, HD value (mean distance) was computed via Distances—Cloud/Mesh Dist under the Tools menu. DSC values were calculated similarly via importing

| Pre-processing parameters of applied filters in MIMICS | | | |
|---|---|---|---|
| **Model no.** | **Filter name** | **Parameter** | **Value** |
| 1 | Binomial blur | Number of iterations | 5 |
| 2 | Curvature flow | Time step | 0.5 |
| | | Number of iterations | 5 |
| 3 | Discrete Gaussian | Gaussian variance | 5 |
| | | Max kernel width | 5 |
| 4 | *Mean | Filter radius | 3 |
| 5 | Median | Filter radius | 3 |
| **Post-processing parameters of applied tools in 3-matic** | | | |
| 6 | *Smooth | Smooth factor | 1 |
| 7 | Wrap | Gap closing | 0.05 |
| | | Smallest detail | 0.5 |
| **Full-processing parameters of both applied filter and tool** | | | |
| 8 | *Mean with *Smooth together | Filter radius | 3 |
| | | Smooth factor | 0.5 |
| *(* = best similarity results).* | | | |

**Table 1.**
*Parameters of each applied filters and tools.*

the reference model and a test model into the 3D workspace of CloudCompare software. The match bounding and fine registration steps were also performed to obtain perfect alignment. After the alignment process, a plugin named as Cork, under the Plugins menu, was utilized to obtain the intersection of both models in terms of volume (cube units). Each volume was also measured by means of the mesh measure volume function under the Edit menu. The DSC value of each model was then calculated to obtain overlapped volume between the two models according to the formula given below ($\alpha$ = total volume of the reference model, $\beta$ = total volume of the compared model, and $\alpha \cap \beta$ = intersection of both models in terms of volume):

$$\mathrm{DSC}\,(\alpha, \beta) = \frac{2\,(\alpha \cap \beta)}{\alpha + \beta} \tag{1}$$

## 3. Results

Wrap tool, binomial blur, and curvature flow filters produce high geometrical errors, while mean filter produces the lowest geometrical error. Furthermore, HD and DSC results of the curvature flow and discrete Gaussian filters are close to mean filter. Smooth tool and mean filter produce almost the same volume of the reference model. However, binomial blur filter and wrap tool generate unacceptably different volumes. Moreover, the DSC results of the both mentioned functions are not overlapping properly. Each result is illustrated in **Table 2**.

Smooth and wrap tools generate undesired mesh structures caused by the noise during the segmentation step in MIMICS. HD results of each test model are illustrated in **Figure 3**.

| HD and DSC results of each test model | | | | | | |
|---|---|---|---|---|---|---|
| **No.** | **Filter-tool name** | **Filter type** | **Model volume (cube units)** | **Max error (%)** | **HD (mm)** | **DSC (0–1)** |
| 1 | Binomial blur | Pre | 80393.9 | 9.502507 | 1.083704 | 0.547654 |
| 2 | Curvature flow | Pre | 81445.2 | 8.31908 | 1.107846 | 0.923381 |
| 3 | Discrete Gaussian | Pre | 81787.5 | 7.933765 | 1.034391 | 0.911621 |
| 4 | Mean | Pre | 82308.1 | 7.347738 | 1.041506 | 0.913479 |
| 5 | Median | Pre | 79867.7 | 10.09483 | 1.043368 | 0.911775 |
| 6 | Smooth | Post | 90480.1 | −1.851286 | 1.185564 | 0.937718 |
| 7 | Wrap | Post | 113,092 | −27.30496 | 0.461971 | 0.871986 |
| 8 | Mean + Smooth | Together | 82231.4 | 7.434077 | 1.041154 | 0.916657 |
| Reference model volume (cube units): 88835.5 | | | | | | |

**Table 2.**
*Results of each applied filters and tools (DSC value: 0 = no overlap, 1 = exact overlap, negative max error values indicate a larger volume than the reference model while positive values mean a lower volume according to the reference model in terms of cube units).*

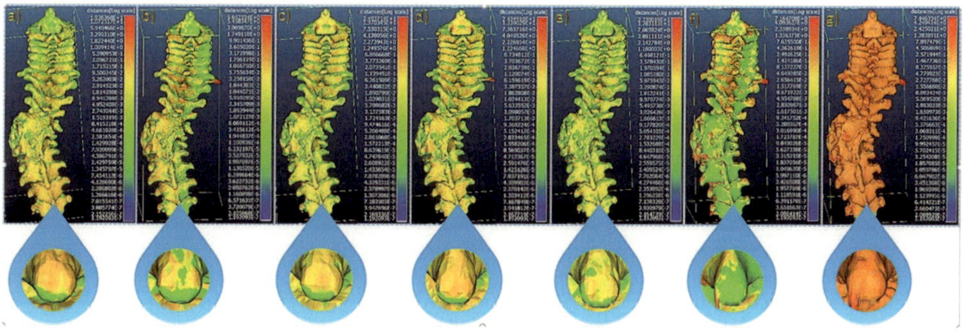

**Figure 3.**
*The intersection of reference model and each generated 3D test model with a local view (a) Reference model and Binomial blur pre-filtered test model, (b) Reference model and Curvature flow pre-filtered test model, (c) Reference model and Discrete gaussian pre-filtered test model, (d) Reference model and Mean pre-filtered test model, (e) Reference model and Median pre-filtered test model, (f) Reference model and Smooth post-filtered test model and (g) Reference model and Wrap post-filtered test model.*

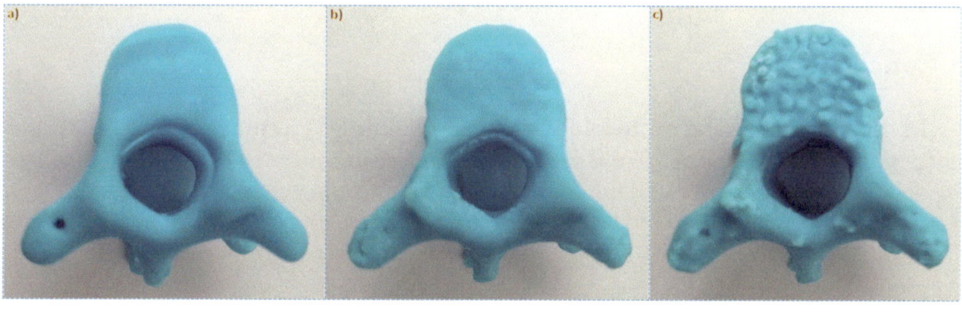


**Figure 4.**
*Results of each produced model. (a) Reference model, (b) Mean filter and (c) Smooth tool.*

The results of the last case given in **Table 2** (mean filter with Smooth tool together) show that increased Smooth provides to obtain better HD and DSC results when compared to the fourth test case (mean filter only). However, the max error is proportionally increased with the Smooth tool. Reference model, mean filter, and Smooth tool results are illustrated in **Figure 4**.

## 4. Discussion

According to the results, binomial blur filter, median filter, and wrap tool are not suitable for surgical planning of a spine model due to the high error percentage in volume. These functions produce misleading information when used alone and may be used with another filter together at lower parametric values. Although Smooth tool provides better DSC result than the curvature flow filter, mesh surface improvement should not be performed by means of this tool only because of the undesired mesh structures caused by the noise. Therefore, a prefilter-like curvature flow, discrete Gaussian, or mean should to be applied on raw DICOM images to filter noise more accurately during the segmentation step, and Smooth tool should to be used at lower values after 3D model reconstruction process. It should be noted that some geometrical errors may not be fixed via 3-matic software and may require a third party software such as Geomagic Design X or Autodesk Meshmixer. On the other hand, fractured or unbounded bone structures may be lost during the noise filtering process. Therefore, some functions such as largest surface selection in MIMICS should not be used in complex cases, and target model should be cleared manually after the 3D reconstruction process. Mesh distribution of the models require to be uniform to perform a healthy DSC calculation. Both reference and compared test models may be processed via optimize mesh tool in Geomagic Design X to achieve uniform mesh distribution on each model.

While software optimizations may be performed to obtain an ideal protocol, improvements may also be applied on used CT device at the beginning for more correct presurgical planning. Devices with more advanced detector structure, which could provide to operate at lower voxels and have high beam quality, may reduce noise on raw data images. For example, it is known that dual energy computed tomography (DECT) is more suitable for tissue segmentation than single-energy computed tomography (SECT) [30]. Besides, some known sources of noise (beam hardening, partial volume effect, etc.) can be reduced by making some adjustments before imaging such as in monochromatic X-ray, reduced beam hardening effect and thin section thickness, and reduced the partial volume effect, which are very important for spine imaging [31, 32]. Additionally, using higher tube current provides sharper image because of the amount of beam delivery to the target tissue. However, high current may not be applied in all cases because of the increased radiation dose given to the patient.

## 5. Conclusion

In this study, an ideal protocol for surgical planning of a spine surgery is defined with measurable accuracy. Thus, success rate of a spine surgery may be increased especially for the severe cases owing to the more accurate preoperative review.

## Acknowledgements

We declare that we have no acknowledgments.

## Author details

Levent Aydin[1], Ozgur Cakir[2], Riza Dilek[3] and Mucahit Ege[1]*

1 Biomedical Device Technology, Istanbul Gedik University, Istanbul, Turkey

2 Department of Radiology, Faculty of Medicine, Kocaeli University, Kocaeli, Turkey

3 Medical Imaging Techniques, Istanbul Gedik University, Istanbul, Turkey

*Address all correspondence to: mucahit.ege@gedik.edu.tr

## References

[1] Choudhry MN, Ahmad Z, Verma R. Adolescent idiopathic scoliosis. The Open Orthopaedics Journal. 2016;**10**:143

[2] Scoliosis—Better Health Channel. 2019. Available from: betterhealth.vic.gov.au/health/ConditionsAndTreatments/scoliosis?viewAsPdf=true [Accessed: June 20, 2019]

[3] Miller MD, Thompson SR, Hart J. Review of orthopaedics. Elsevier Health Sciences; 2012. p. 1

[4] Treating Scoliosis. 2019. Available from: https://www.treatingscoliosis.com/infographics/scoliosis-by-the-numbers/ [Accessed: June 20, 2019]

[5] Napierkowski DB. Scoliosis: A case study in an adolescent boy. Orthopaedic Nursing. 2007;**26**(3):147-155

[6] Grauers A, Einarsdottir E, Gerdhem P. Genetics and pathogenesis of idiopathic scoliosis. Scoliosis and Spinal Disorders. 2016;**11**(1):45

[7] University of Maryland School of Medicine. 2019. Available from: https://www.umms.org/ummc/health-services/orthopedics/services/spine/patient-guides/complications-spine-surgery [Accessed: June 20, 2019]

[8] Rengier F, Mehndiratta A, Von Tengg-Kobligk H, et al. 3d printing based on imaging data: Review of medical applications. International Journal of Computer Assisted Radiology and Surgery. 2010;**5**(4):335-341

[9] Kido T, Kurata A, Higashino H, et al. Cardiac imaging using 256-detector row four-dimensional CT: Preliminary clinical report. Radiation Medicine. 2007;**25**(1):38-44

[10] Palau JR. Three-dimensional planning in craniomaxillofacial surgery. International Journal of Oral and Maxillofacial Surgery. 2017;**46**:46

[11] Chae MP, Rozen WM, McMenamin PG, et al. Emerging applications of bedside 3d printing in plastic surgery. Frontiers in Surgery. 2015;**2**:25

[12] Aydin L, Kucuk S. A method for more accurate fea results on a medical device developed by 3d technologies. Polymers for Advanced Technologies. 2018;**29**(8):2281-2286

[13] Kurenov SN, Ionita C, Sammons D, et al. Three-dimensional printing to facilitate anatomic study, device development, simulation, and planning in thoracic surgery. The Journal of Thoracic and Cardiovascular Surgery. 2015;**149**(4):973-979

[14] Wallace GG, Cornock RC, O'Connell CD, et al. 3d Bioprinting: Printing Parts for Bodies. Vol. 1566. ARC Centre of Excellence for Electromaterials Science; 2014. p. 1. ISBN 978-0-646-92867-8

[15] Dawood A, Marti BM, Sauret-Jackson V, et al. 3d printing in dentistry. British Dental Journal. 2015;**219**(11):521

[16] Zhu W, Qu X, Zhu J, et al. Direct 3d bioprinting of prevascularized tissue constructs with complex microarchitecture. Biomaterials. 2017;**124**:106-115

[17] Murphy SV, Atala A. 3d bioprinting of tissues and organs. Nature Biotechnology. 2014;**32**(8):773

[18] Mulford JS, Babazadeh S, Mackay N. Three-dimensional printing in orthopaedic surgery: Review of current and future applications. ANZ Journal of Surgery. 2016;**86**(9):648-653

[19] Samset E, Schmalstieg D, Vander Sloten J, et al. Augmented Reality in Surgical Procedures. Human Vision and Electronic Imaging XIII ; 2008. p. 68060K

[20] Modabber A, Ayoub N, Bock A, et al. Medial approach for minimally-invasive harvesting of a deep circumflex iliac artery flap for reconstruction of the jaw using virtual surgical planning and cad/cam technology. British Journal of Oral and Maxillofacial Surgery. 2017;**55**(9):946-951

[21] Guo HC, Wang Y, Dai J, et al. Application of 3d printing in the surgical planning of hypertrophic obstructive cardiomyopathy and physician-patient communication: A preliminary study. Journal of Thoracic Disease. 2018;**10**(2):867

[22] Starosolski ZA, Kan JH, Rosenfeld SD, et al. Application of 3-d printing (rapid prototyping) for creating physical models of pediatric orthopedic disorders. Pediatric Radiology. 2014;**44**(2):216-221

[23] Flügge TV, Nelson K, Schmelzeisen R, et al. Three-dimensional plotting and printing of an implant drilling guide: Simplifying guided implant surgery. Journal of Oral and Maxillofacial Surgery. 2013;**71**(8):1340-1346

[24] Egger J, Kapur T, Fedorov A, et al. GBM volumetry using the 3d slicer medical image computing platform. Scientific Reports. 2013;**3**:1364

[25] Egger J, Gall M, Tax A, et al. Interactive reconstructions of cranial 3d implants under mevislab as an alternative to commercial planning software. PLoS One. 2017;**12**(3):e0172694

[26] Deeley MA, Chen A, Datteri R, et al. Comparison of manual and automatic segmentation methods for brain structures in the presence of space-occupying lesions: A multi-expert study. Physics in Medicine & Biology. 2011;**56**(14):4557

[27] Taha AA, Hanbury A. An efficient algorithm for calculating the exact hausdorff distance. IEEE Transactions on Pattern Analysis and Machine Intelligence. 2015;**37**(11):2153-2163

[28] Bulbul A, Capin T, Lavoué G, et al. Assessing visual quality of 3-d polygonal models. IEEE Signal Processing Magazine. 2011;**28**(6):80-90

[29] Cloud Compare. 2019. Available from: https://www.cloudcompare.org/doc/qCC/CloudCompare%20v2.6.1%20-%20User%20manual.pdf [Accessed: June 20, 2019]

[30] Nora H. Dual energy CT as an alternative for ion radiotherapy treatment planning [doctoral dissertation]. Germany: Combined Faculties for the Natural Sciences and for Mathematics of the Ruperto-Carola University of Heidelberg; 2014

[31] Torikoshi M, Tsunoo T, Sasaki M. Electron density measurement with dual-energy x-ray ct using synchrotron radiation. Physics in Medicine & Biology. 2003;**48**(5):673-685

[32] Kemerink GJ. The nonlinear partial volume effect and computed tomography densitometry of foam and lung. Medical Physics. 1995;**22**(9):1445-1450

Section 5

# Robotic Urologic Surgery

Chapter 6

# Ureteropelvic Junction Obstruction: Robot-Assisted Pyeloplasty

*Pietro Diana, Paolo Casale, Alberto Rosario Saita, Giovanni Lughezzani and Nicolomaria Buffi*

## Abstract

The standard treatment of ureteropelvic junction obstruction (UPJO) is represented by the Anderson-Hynes dismembered pyeloplasty, even if different approaches, both surgical and endoscopic, have been described. Robot-assisted pyeloplasty (RP) is a feasible and safe approach. The indications for the robotic approach remain the same as those for the laparoscopic or open pyeloplasty. Every patient with symptomatic UPJO, or with decreasing renal function in the presence of UPJO, should undergo RP. The transperitoneal, retroperitoneal, and transmesocolic approaches are described focusing on advantages and disadvantages of each approach. Robot-assisted pyeloplasty has excellent success rates for relief of obstruction and very low peri- and post-operative morbidity. The robotic surgical technique maintains the advantages of laparoscopic surgery providing a more precise manipulation and visualization, and a faster learning curve. Comparative studies are reported to confront the different techniques. Secondary minimally invasive pyeloplasty is obviously a more challenging procedure due to the fibrosis and the adhesions formed after the previous surgery. Newer techniques and indications such as the employment of buccal mucosal graft, the single port approach, and indocyanine green injection are described. Tips and tricks to keep in mind during this kind of procedure are listed in order to report our experience in this setting.

**Keywords:** ureteropelvic junction obstruction, robot-assisted pyeloplasty, robotic surgery

## 1. Introduction

The standard treatment of ureteropelvic junction obstruction (UPJO) is represented by the Anderson-Hynes dismembered pyeloplasty, even if different approaches, both surgical and endoscopic, have been described.

The Anderson-Hynes dismembered pyeloplasty was first described in 1993 by Schuessler et al. [1], and the laparoscopic approach has become the gold standard in alternative to the open approach as the long-term outcomes are comparable between the two techniques with success rates from 90 to >95% [2–5]. However, laparoscopic pyeloplasty, both through a transperitoneal and a retroperitoneal approach, remains a challenging procedure and it requires high proficiency in laparoscopic skills especially due to the reconstructive part. In fact, even in large series of referral centers, the operative time remains extensive.

The robot-assisted laparoscopic approach overcomes the limits of conventional laparoscopy thanks to the three-dimensional vision, increased tools dexterity, and greater precision. Therefore, considering the reconstruction skills needed for intracorporeal suturing, dismembered pyeloplasty most benefits from the robotic assistance.

Robotic pyeloplasty (RP) using the Da Vinci (Intuitive Surgical, Inc., Sunnyvale, CA, USA) system has been first described by Gettman et al. in 2002 [6], reporting perioperative outcomes of 9 patients treated with robotic transperitoneal pyeloplasty for UPJO.

### 1.1 Indications to robotic dismembered pyeloplasty

The indications for the robotic approach remain the same as those for the laparoscopic or open pyeloplasty. Every patient with symptomatic UPJO, or with decreasing renal function in the presence of UPJO, should undergo RP. Additionally, patients that failed primary treatment, the robotic approach could be considered.

The diagnostic workout mirrors the one for the open and laparoscopic approach. The patients should undergo diuretic MAG4 renogram and CT scan to evaluate the anatomy, such as the presence of a crossing vessel and the eventual presence of renal calculi to plan the surgical strategy accordingly.

## 2. Surgical strategies

### 2.1 Transperitoneal approach for robot-assisted pyeloplasty

#### *2.1.1 Operating room setup*

The patient is placed at a 60° full flank position exposing upward the affected side. The two arms are placed on an arm board and alongside the patient's flank, respectively. Both legs are fully extended and the upper one is abducted with one or two pillows placed in between. Extension of the operating table is performed breaking the patient's flack midway between the iliac crest and the costal margin to obtain a broader operating field (**Figure 1**).

The OR setup can be seen in **Figure 2**. Anesthesia takes position at the head of the patient. The robotic cart is coming from the patient's back.

#### *2.1.2 Robotic ports*

The optic trocar is placed at the level of the umbilicus, for esthetic reasons, or on pararectal line for obese patients always at the umbilical level. Trocars of 12 or 8 mm are used for the Si and Xi DaVinci system, respectively. Either a 30° or a 0° camera is employed depending on the operator preference. The two operative robotic ports are positioned at the midpoint between the anterior superior iliac spine and the umbilicus and on the pararectal line at least 1 cm below the costal arch. The 5-mm assistant port is placed cranially in respect to the camera port at the midpoint between the umbilicus and the xiphoid process (**Figure 3**).

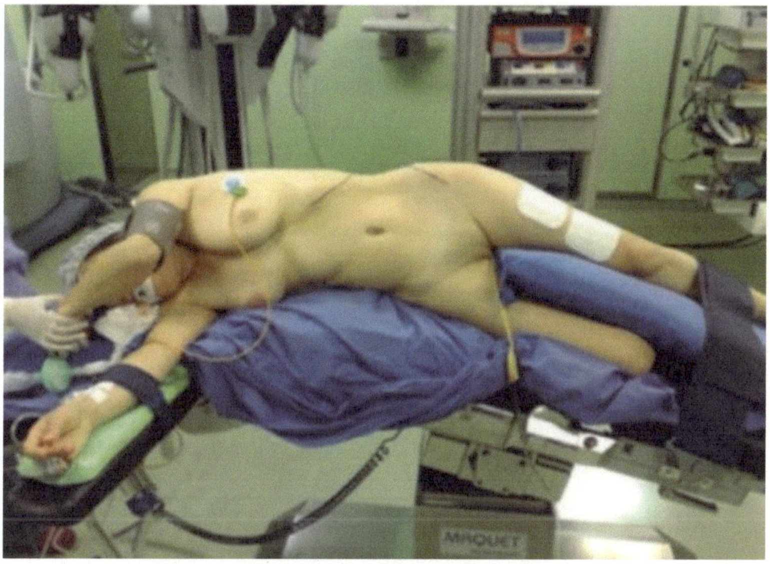

**Figure 1.**
*Patient's position for transperitoneal robotic pyeloplasty.*

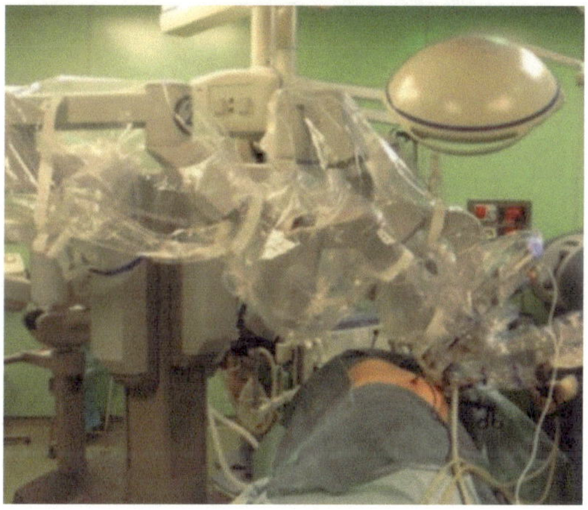

**Figure 2.**
*Operating theater setup for transperitoneal robotic pyeloplasty.*

### *2.1.3 Procedure step-by-step*

After the medialization of the colon, on the right side, the overlying Gerota's fascia is incised, while on the right side, the white line of Toldt is incised and the left colon is mobilized medially. Despite the side, the target structures (the ureter, the dilated renal pelvis, and eventually the aberrant crossing vessels) are exposed. The ureter can be visualized by following the psoas muscle medially starting from the lower pole of the kidney. Any crossing vessels are identified and preserved. The UPJ is fully mobilized using both blunt and sharp dissection. Bipolar fenestrated forceps and monopolar scissors are employed in this phase.

When the UPJ is isolated and the obstruction is identified, section of the ureter is performed. In case of a severe dilation of the pelvis, the redundant portion should be excised. The presence of renal calculi in the renal pelvis implies its removal with the employment of a flexible cystoscope. The ureter is then spatulated

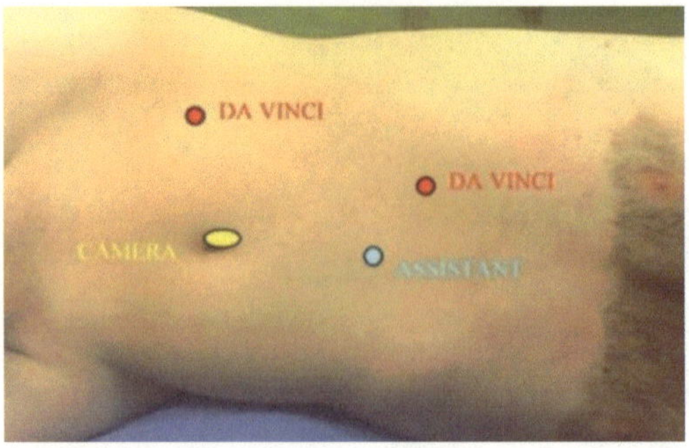


**Figure 3.**
*Port placement for transperitoneal robotic pyeloplasty.*

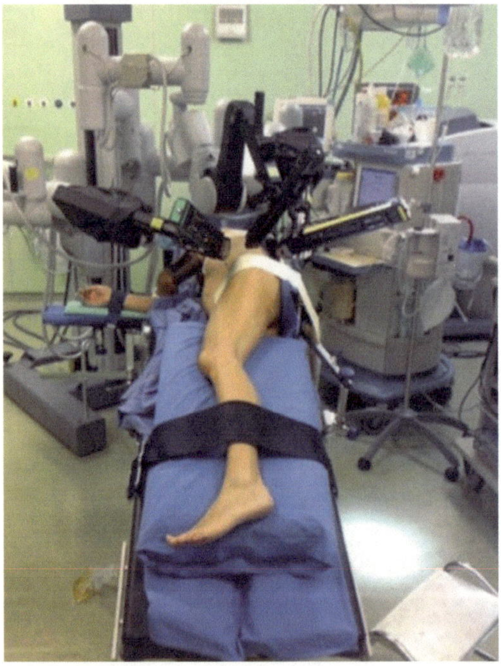

**Figure 4.**
*Patient's position for retroperitoneal robotic pyeloplasty.*

longitudinally up to the visualization of healthy tissue; the pyeloplasty is then performed according to the Anderson-Hynes technique. Two 4-0 Vicryl running sutures are preferred for the anastomosis, one for the posterior and the other for the anterior plate using a robotic needle driver.

In the case of a crossing vessel, a dismembered pyeloplasty is performed with anterior transposition of the ureteral anastomosis in respect to the blood vessels.

## 2.2 Retroperitoneal approach for robot-assisted pyeloplasty

### *2.2.1 Operating room setup*

As seen in **Figure 4**, the patient is placed in a full flank position with the operating table extended to maximize the operating field. The robotic system is placed in order to enter the arms anteriorly of 25–30° in respect to the head of the patient.

*2.2.2 Robotic ports*

A retroperitoneal access is performed at the level of the tip of the 12th rib. A Balloon expander or other cost-effective alternatives (such as a finger of sterile gloves tied to a trocar and filled with saline water) [7] are used to create a working space in the retroperitoneal fat. The two operative ports are positioned at the crossover of the 12th rib and the erector spinae muscle and at the level of the anterior axillary line 6–8 cm cranially to the iliac crest, respectively. A 5-mm trocar for the assistant is positioned along the erector spinae muscle, cranially to the iliac crest (**Figure 5**).

*2.2.3 Procedure step-by-step*

The Gerota's fascia is excised and the UPJ is exposed. The plasty mirrors the transperitoneal approach.

### 2.3 Transperitoneal versus retroperitoneal access

Cestari et al. [5] reported outcomes of 36 and 19 patients who underwent retroperitoneal and transperitoneal robotic pyeloplasty, respectively. They stated that either the transperitoneal or retroperitoneal approach is feasible and safe, comparable in terms of operative time, estimated blood loss, and postoperative complications. No cases of conversion were reported.

Regarding the transperitoneal approach, given the wider working space, it is usually preferred in case of a wide renal pelvis (>6 cm), presence of pelvic calculi, crossing vessels, renal malformations (i.e., horseshoe kidney), or pelvic kidney.

The advantage of the retroperitoneal access comprehends a direct exposure of the UPJ without the opening of the peritoneal cavity and minimizing intraperitoneal organs injury. However, the lack of familiar anatomical reference structures and a narrow operative space are limitations of this approach. Additionally, using a retroperitoneal access gives the possibility to manage conservatively urinary fistulas, since urine will remain in the retroperitoneal cavity.

### 2.4 Transmesocolic approach for the left robot-assisted pyeloplasty

Gupta et al. reported in 2009 the transmesocolic access for the left UPJO [8] through an incision of the mesocolon. This approach allows the operator to access directly the left renal pelvis and UPJ without mobilizing the descending colon.

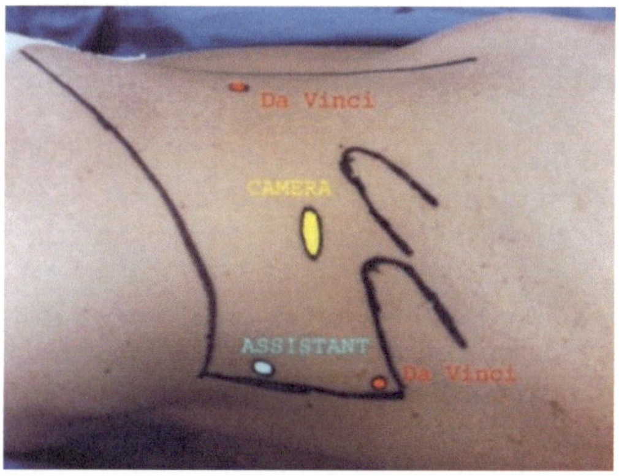


**Figure 5.**
*Port placement for retroperitoneal robotic pyeloplasty.*

The best candidates for this approach are young thin patients, with a large renal pelvis. In the case of renal calculi or either previous or present history of a complicated ureteropelvic junction obstruction, a transperitoneal approach might be the access of choice.

The transmesocolic approach brings advantages such as a shorter mean operative time and hospital stay, and a faster bowel peristalsis recovery as described in the literature [9, 10].

## 2.5 Ureteral stenting in robot-assisted pyeloplasty

A ureteral stent is necessary to protect the anastomosis from high renal intrapelvic pressure. Therefore, a ureteral stent is usually placed during the procedure either in a retrograde or anterograde fashion.

Retrograde stent placement is performed in the operating room before the procedure. A retrograde pyelogram during the double J position can exclude any other ureteric abnormalities. However, it is more time-consuming as the patient is before proceeding with the surgery; moreover, stenting results in the collapse of the renal pelvis, making the identification of the UPJ stricture more difficult.

Anterograde stenting consists in putting the ureteral double-J stent during the pyeloplasty. In this way, the collapse of the renal pelvis is avoided. Usually, a hydrophilic guidewire and a 5-Fr ureteral catheter are inserted through the 5-mm trocar after suturing the posterior aspect of the anastomosis. The guidewire and the catheter are pushed within the ureter with a robotic grasper or a needle driver down to the bladder. Then, the ureteral catheter is removed and the double-J stent is placed onto the guidewire. After the stent placement, the anterior aspect of the anastomosis is completed. This technique is safe, feasible and time-saving [11]. Disadvantage consists in the blind placement of the stent. Correct stent placement can be assured by fluoroscopy or an abdominal X-Ray; another technique has been reported by Rodrigues et al. [12] using methylene blue to fill the bladder and its appearance through the stent holes as an indicator of correct positioning.

Gaitonde et al. [13] used a cystoscopically placed ureteropelvic junction occlusion catheter positioned along with a marked Foley urethral catheter to display the distance required to accurately position the lower coil of the stent into the bladder. The Foley and the occlusion balloon are prepared and after pyelotomy, the balloon is deflated, and the occlusion catheter is withdrawn into the proximal ureter. After completing the posterior aspect of the anastomosis, a guidewire is inserted through the catheter and grasped at the kidney pelvis. The occlusion catheter is then removed and the stent pushed along the guidewire up to the renal pelvis. The distal end of the stent pusher was advanced until the calibrated mark of the Foley catheter appears to ensure the correct positioning of the distal coil in the bladder.

Fiori et al. reported flexible pneumocystoscopy as safe and feasible in placing a retrograde ureteral stent in the setting of laparoscopic pyeloplasty. In this way, the patient can be placed directly on the flank position and the reconstruction can proceed [14].

Studies comparing retrograde versus an anterograde stenting approach have been done. For all the studies, the setting is the laparoscopic pyeloplasty. Anterograde stenting is quicker; however, retrograde stenting appears to ensure a higher success rate in correct stent placement [15–18]. Stentless pyeloplasty has also been reported; however, very few and conflicting reports evaluate the safety and the efficacy of a stentless approach [19–21].

### 2.6 Postoperative management

Patient's mobilization and feeding can start postoperative day 1. The bladder catheter is usually removed on postoperative day 2 and the drain the following day if the output is less than 50–70 mL; patients are discharged on the same day.

Stent removal occurs after 4 weeks postoperatively. On the same occasion, urinalysis, urine culture, and abdominal ultrasound can be prescribed in order to assess the short-term operative outcome.

Patients are then evaluated at 6 and 12 months with urinalysis, urine culture, MAG3 renogram, and URO-CT scan.

## 3. Surgical outcomes

Robot-assisted pyeloplasty has excellent success rates for relief of obstruction and very low peri- and post-operative morbidity. The robotic surgical technique maintains the advantages of laparoscopic surgery, providing a more precise manipulation and visualization and a faster learning curve.

Several methods and variables may be adopted to define resolution of the obstruction including radiology and nuclear medicine tests (renogram, intravenous pyelogram, or ultrasound), symptom resolution, and laboratory analysis.

Ultrasound can lead to an incorrect interpretation of obstruction resolution as the persistent residual hydronephrosis can be seen for months or longer after the procedure.

Renal scintigraphy is widely recognized as the best noninvasive imaging modality to define the obstruction and it is employed in the evaluation of the postoperative outcomes.

The first experience with robot-assisted Anderson-Hynes pyeloplasty was published by Getmann et al. in 2002 [6]. The authors reported outcomes of 9 consecutive patients treated with transperitoneal robotic pyeloplasty. No surgical conversion was reported and 1 patient underwent an open surgery in the second place because of a urinary fistula. Favorable outcome for all patients was reported at 4 months follow-up.

Patel published a 50-patient series reaching 100% of success rate. Operative success was defined by a negative MAG3 renography. The authors stated that this technique offers short-term efficacy and a very low rate of complications, with a quick learning curve [22].

Mufarrij et al. reported a multi-institutional series of 140 patients, with 29 months follow-up, including both primary and secondary UPJO. The success rate reached the 96% of the cases and recurrence was reported in six cases. Complication rate was 7.1% and, postoperatively, double-J stent migration was the most common complication. As for minor complications, fever was the most frequently described [23].

Schwentner et al. published in 2007. A large series of 92 patients, 80 with primary obstruction and 12 with secondary ones, were described. The follow-up reached up to 40 months and the success rate was 96%. In the secondary obstruction, the arm failure rate after RP was slightly higher [24].

The optimal results of the robotic procedure were confirmed in another multi-institutional large series of 169 patients, both primary and secondary obstructions being taken into account. The success rate reached 97.6% with 39 months follow-up. The mean estimated blood loss (EBL) was around 50 mL and the complication rate was 6.6% [25].

| Authors | Number of patients | Tranperitoneal vs. retroperitoneal approach | Operative time (min) | Conversion rate (%) | Complication rate (%) | Hospital stay (days) | Follow-up (months) |
|---|---|---|---|---|---|---|---|
| Patel [22] | 50 | Transperitoneal | 122 | 0 | 32 | 1.1 | 11.7 |
| Olsen et al. [30] | 67 | Retroperitoneal | 146 | 1.5 | 17.9 | 2 | 12.1 |
| Schwentner et al. [24] | 92 | Transperitoneal | 108 | 0 | NA | 4.6 | 39.1 |
| Mufarrij et al. [23] | 140 | Transperitoneal | 217 | 0 | 10 | 2.1 | 29 |
| Guptal et al. [31] | 86 | Transperitoneal | 121 | 2.3 | 9.3 | 2.5 | 13.6 |
| Minnillo et al. [28] | 155 | Transperitoneal | 198.5 | 0 | 11 | 1.95 | 31.7 |
| Etafy et al. [32] | 61 | Transperitoneal | 335 | 0 | 11.4 | 2 | 18 |
| Sivaraman et al. [25] | 168 | Transperitoneal | 134.9 | 0 | 6.6 | 1.5 | 39 |
| Buffi et al. [33] | 145 | Both | 120 | 2.8 | 8.3 | 4.7 | 24 |

**Table 1.**
*Comparative studies (more than 50 patients)*

Cestari et al. reported that both the retro- and transperitoneal RPs were safe and these were the feasible procedures with a low morbidity rate with an overall success rate of 96% [5].

Overall, the outcomes of the procedure have been defined as excellent and reproducible [22, 25, 26], with durable results [24].

The success rate reported [27] is high (81–100%), with reintervention rates between 0 and 13.1%. Operative times are more variable, ranging from 105 to 335 min. They concluded RP to be a safe procedure with a reproducible high rate of successful outcomes, low conversion rates (0–4.8%), complication rates (2–17.9%), and a limited EBL.

Outcomes of RP in the pediatric population have been largely described in the literature. Minnillo et al. published the largest series, assessing 155 pediatric patients undergoing RP; a success rate of 96% with a 3% of failure rate was reported [28].

A recent meta-analysis of comparative studies in the pediatric population showed no difference in success rate between robotic and conventional laparoscopic pyeloplasty [29] with an overall success rate of 99.3% and 96.9%, respectively, with no significant difference between the two approaches. Complication and reoperation rates were comparable between the two approaches. The length of hospitalization was significantly shorter for the robotic group (**Table 1**).

A recent multi-institutional study [34] reported 407 pediatric cases treated with robotic pyeloplasty and found a complication rate of 13.8%. No high-grade complications were reported (Clavien Dindo IV or V).

### 3.1 Comparative studies

Autorino et al. published a meta-analysis that demonstrates no statistically significant difference in terms of success and complication rates between minimally invasive and open approach in the adult population; however, the minimally invasive approaches provides a shorter hospital stay compared to open surgery [27].

Basatac et al. [35] confirmed the significant decrease in the length of hospital stay, estimated blood loss, earlier drainage removal, and the decrease of the need for painkillers. In terms of success rates, intraoperative complications, and conversions, no significant differences were found.

Basatac et al. described a shorter time for robotic surgery although considering exclusively the console time. Hanske et al. [36], when evaluating a large number of patients undergoing minimally invasive versus open, reports a statistically significant difference in the percentage of patients requiring prolonged operation time (<236 min): 29.6% for minimally invasive pyeloplasty versus 15.3% for open pyeloplasty.

## 4. Role of robotic approach in the management of recurrent ureteropelvic junction obstruction

The robotic approach is feasible, safe, and effective for treating recurrent obstruction [33]. Secondary minimally invasive pyeloplasty is obviously a more challenging procedure due to the fibrosis and the adhesions formed after the previous surgery. The precise movements with the robotic assistance and the amplified vision provide higher precision, thus, a bloodless dissection and a higher quality of the suture above all in complex patients.

RP in the treatment of secondary obstructions in pediatric series is reported with data from small series of patients. No comparative prospective studies were ever reported.

Thom et al. found that nine secondary robotic procedures done at their center required longer operative time with an increased blood loss and failure rate (22%) [37]. Atug et al. show data from 7 patients undergoing redo RP. The outcomes were compared with data from a series of 37 patients that underwent RP for primary ureteropelvic junction obstruction. Mean operative time was 60 min longer in the secondary RP group. However, EBL, hospital stay, and overall success were comparable [38].

Hemal et al. described the outcomes of 9 patients (mean age: 16.4 year) treated for secondary UPJO after failure of a previous open pyeloplasty and additionally failed endoscopic pyelotomy. All patients were treated robotically and reported clinical resolution of symptoms and no sign of residual obstruction at postoperative renal scan [39].

Data from a series of 20 patients treated for secondary obstruction were published. Redo RP resulted successful in 94% of cases and the procedure was reported as feasible and safe [40].

Another series of 16 pediatric patients affected by secondary ureteropelvic junction obstruction is reported by Lindgren et al. [41]. These patients underwent redo RP following prior intervention, in specific, 12 underwent previous open surgeries and 4 RP. Redo RP and redo robotic ureterocalicostomy were performed in 13 and 3 patients, respectively. Overall resolution of symptoms was 100%, and radiographic test resolution or improvement was reported in 88% of cases. None of the patients needed further surgical treatment at an intermediate-term follow-up.

## 5. Single-site robot-assisted pyeloplasty

The treatment of UPJO is frequently performed in young patients. Thus, besides the resolution of the obstruction, the cosmetic result represents a crucial point in this population. Laparoendoscopic single site (LESS) pyeloplasty has been thought to reach this kind of goal [41, 42].

LESS is a complex approach, particularly due to suturing, even for urologists with an extended experience. This is due to the loss of instrument triangulation and instrument clashing and to the reduced visibility and maneuverability associated with the coaxial orientation of instruments and of the laparoscope. The robotic technology minimizes the limitations associated with laparoendoscopic single site.

Robotic laparoendoscopic single site (R-LESS) pyeloplasty technique is performed with the use of a 2.5 cm umbilical incision. Through this the single site port is inserted and the robot arms are connected (**Figure 6**) [43]. The GelPort system, introduced by a 3–5 cm umbilical incision, has also been employed to perform robotic LESS pyeloplasty [44] (**Figure 7**).

Data from a multicenter series of 30 cases reported the feasibility and safety of R-LESS pyeloplasty in highly selected patients. Only 2 patients were converted into a classic laparoscopic or robot-assisted approach. In three cases, an additional 3 mm trocar was needed. Success rate, at 13 months follow up, was comparable to rates reported in conventional robotic studies.

Exclusion criteria for this approach are a body mass index (BMI) >30 kg/m$^2$, previous surgical procedure, an extremely dilated kidney pelvis (i.e., pelvis diameter > 6 cm), complicated ureteropelvic junction obstruction with calculi, pelvic kidney, and horseshoe kidney [45, 46].

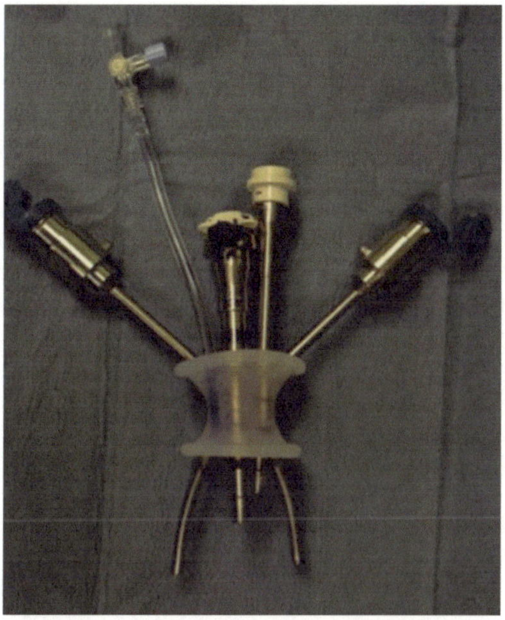

**Figure 6.**
*Da Vinci single site.*

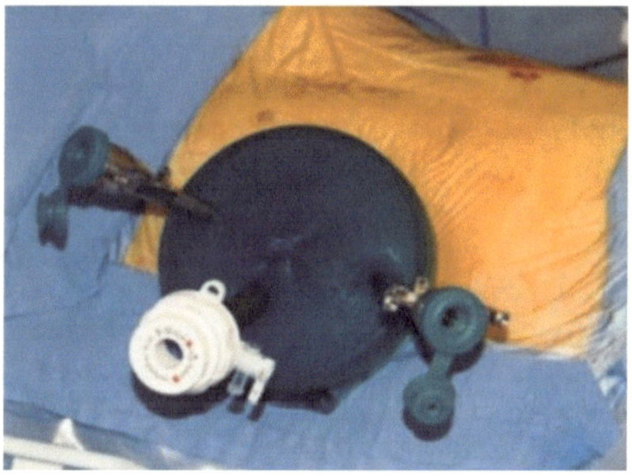

**Figure 7.**
*The GelPort system.*

R-LESS pyeloplasty is considered as a feasible and reproducible procedure in selected cases offering shorter hospitalization. Real advantages compared to the standard robot-assisted pyeloplasty are still to be shown in terms of operative outcome.

## 6. Buccal mucosal graft in pyeloplasty

Management of recurrent UPJO has lower success rate compared to primary treatment. Redo pyeloplasty can be challenging due to scar tissue and fibrosis that lead to larger resections to fin healthy and well-vascularized tissue for reanastomosis. Buccal mucosal grafts (BMG), already in use for ureteral reconstruction, have been proposed in UPJO refractory to surgery and endoscopic treatment [47].

The procedure consists in identifying the UPJO and dissecting longitudinally the anterior aspect of the stenosis. The incision is carried 1 cm proximally and distally to the stricture to ensure exposure of healthy tissue. 8-Fr double-J ureteral stents is placed robotically without the use of fluoroscopy. Single buccal graft is then harvested from the right inner cheek avoiding to compromise the Stensen ducts. The graft is placed as an anterior anastomotic onlay, over the ureteral and UPJ defect, with two 4-0 Vicryl sutures in a running fashion. The repair and entire surgical fields are wrapped in omentum after confirming the anastomoses are watertight with retrograde filling of the urinary collecting systems with methylene blue.

Although a handful of cases have been reported, it is a feasible and safe technique in both a pediatric and adult population. In the two studies, 3 and 2 patients were reported and a complete resolution of symptoms with a stable or improved ultrasound was seen at a median follow-up of 10 and 7 months, respectively. No postoperative complications were reported [48, 49].

## 7. The role of indocyanine green in redo pyeloplasty

The use of intraureteral injection indocyanine green (ICG) dye and subsequent visualization under near infra-red fluorescence (NIRF) has been used to facilitate robotic ureteral identification and reconstruction by aiding in rapid and accurate identification of the stricture margins. This can be particularly useful in case of recurrent UPJ interventions since the presence of fibrotic tissue may be a challenge to the surgeon [50, 51].

The procedure consists in inserting a 6-Fr ureteral catheter into the diseased ureter and 10 ml of ICG is injected retrogradely into the lumen, above and below the level of stenosis, and NIRF is used to guide our dissection; healthy tissue appears bright green and fibrotic, less perfused tissue, since it loses its transparency, appears darker giving precise localization of the proximal and distal stricture margins (**Figure 8**). Step-by-step procedure is shown in **Figures 9–15**.

Several series were published proving that the intraureteral injection of ICG is reproducible, safe, easy to perform, and involves minimal additional costs. All cases were clinically and radiographically successful, and no patient has required a repeat operation for stricture recurrence [50].

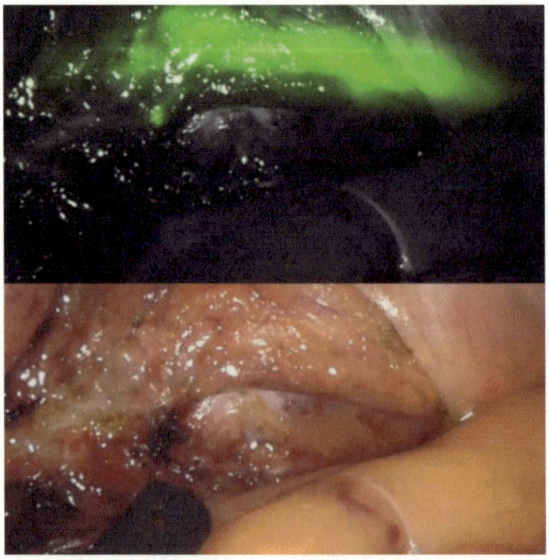

**Figure 8.**
*Intraureteral injection of indocyanine green in a redo pyeloplasty.*

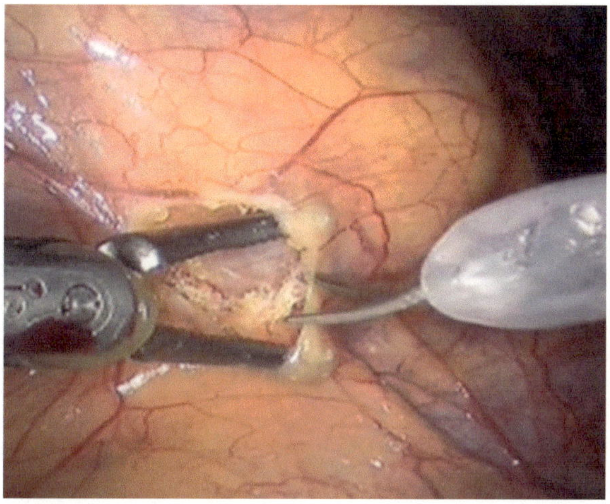

**Figure 9.**
*Peritoneal incision.*

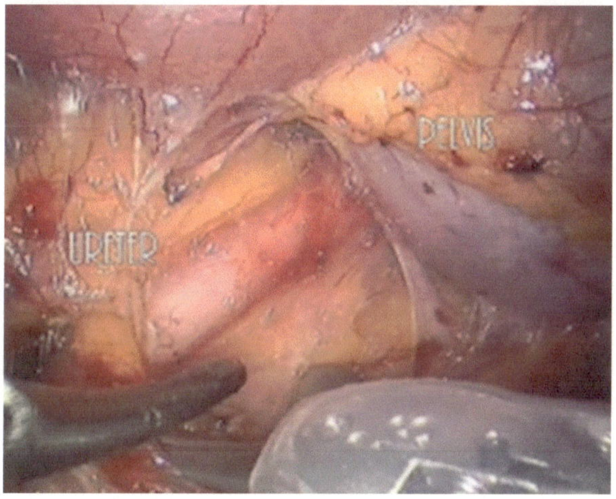


**Figure 10.**
*Structures isolation.*

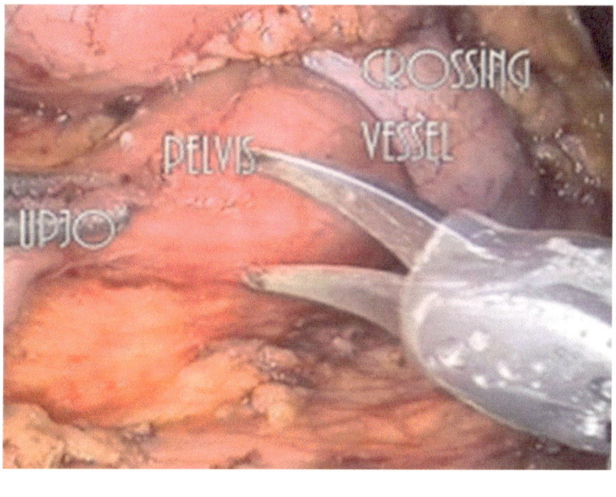


**Figure 11.**
*Exposure of structures.*

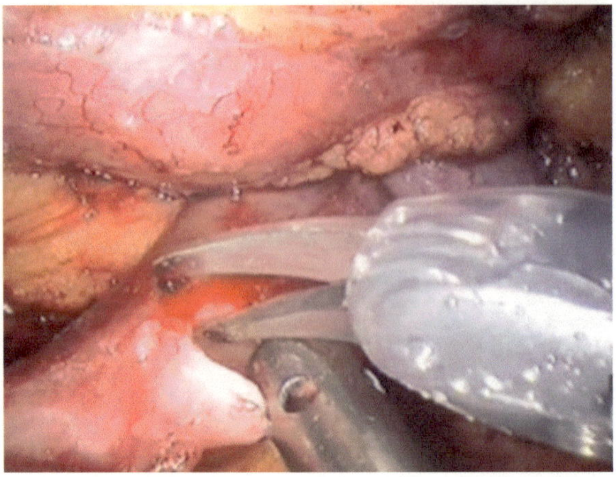

**Figure 12.**
*Ureteral Incision.*

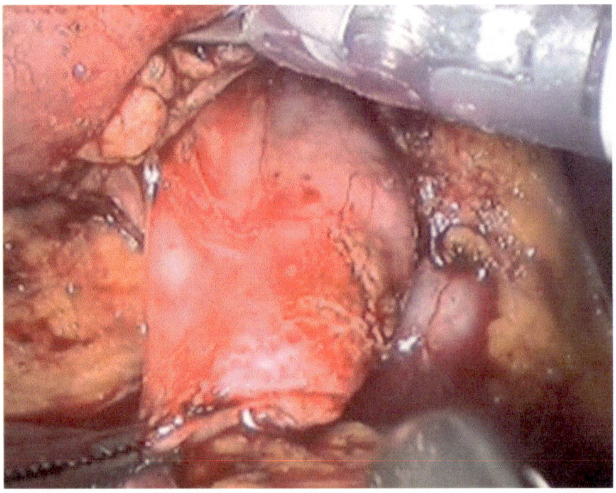

**Figure 13.**
*Decrossing of the renal pelvis.*

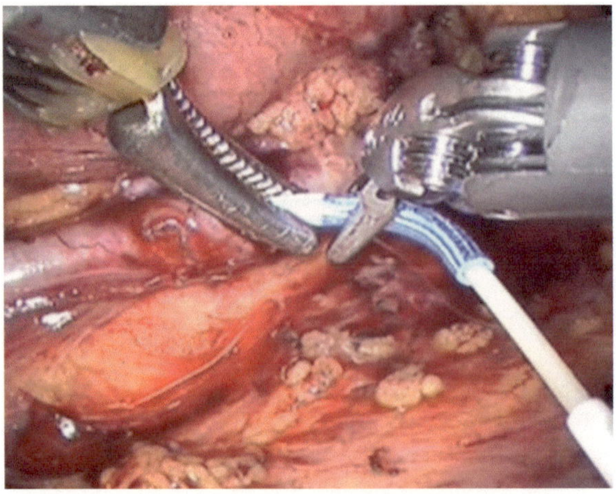

**Figure 14.**
*Anterograde ureteral stenting.*

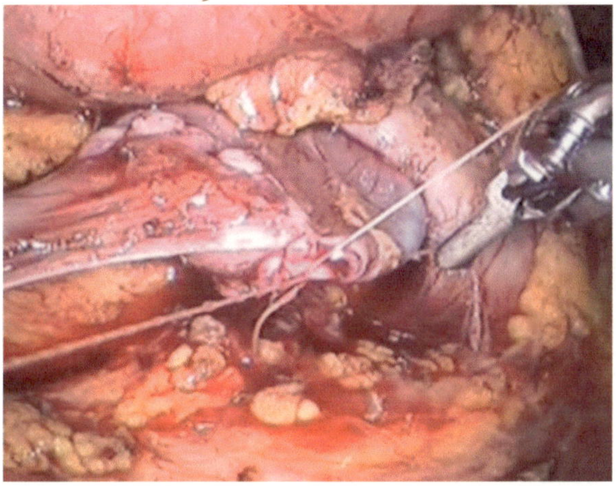

**Figure 15.**
*Anastomosis.*

## 8. Tips and tricks to approach robot-assisted pyeloplasty

Here, the steps where we think it is most important not to underestimate are described.

First of all particular attention should be given to the ports placement; although, it could sound trivial if you have a wrong port positioning the surgery might result challenging and the failure rate and risk of complications increase. During the diagnostic workout, a CT scan is performed not only to check for the presence of renal stones and a crossing vessel but also to understand the anatomy and the relationship of the kidney with the renal pelvis. The kidney can be ectopic, also called pelvic, and this would change the trocars placement. UPJO incidence reaches up to 22–37% of ectopic kidneys [52]. The camera port is still placed at the umbilicus level. The two operative robotic ports are positioned on the homolateral side as affected kidney 8 cm apart laterally on the same line as the camera and the 5-mm assistant port is positioned at the distal third on the line between the superior anterior iliac crest and the umbilicus.

Ureteral isolation is also fundamental for reducing the peri-operative risks and to better manage the ureter during the reconstruction phase. Several are the challenging scenarios where the importance of the ureteral isolation cannot be overstated. In the redo pyeloplasty, the fibrotic tissue makes both the identification and the handling of the structures more difficult and the risk of failure might increases if the ureter is not well isolated; as said the use of intraureteral ICG can help during this phase. Other scenarios can be encountered in the case of extra-rotated kidneys and intrarenal pelvis where the structures can be hidden and, in these cases, a partial isolation of the kidney and marker stitches can be placed to better expose the structures and a larger surgical field.

It is important not to underestimate the presence of calculi in the renal pelvis. In these cases, a flexible cystoscope can be inserted though one of the robotic trocars and consequently inserted into the real pelvis through a small incision previously performed. This is important as it allows stone extraction or even lithotripsy avoiding spilling of water into the peritoneal cavity.

Finally, the ureteropelvic anastomosis if one of the most crucial phases of this kind of surgery as it is fundamental to have a continent anastomosis to avoid urinary fistulas, but is as important not to have an over tight suturing that would create again a stricture of the junction. Barbed sutures are advised as the barbs on its surface penetrate inside the tissue and lock them into place enabling the surgeon to adjust the tightness of the anastomosis.

## Author details

Pietro Diana[1,2], Paolo Casale[1], Alberto Rosario Saita[1,2], Giovanni Lughezzani[1,2] and Nicolomaria Buffi[1,2*]

1 Department of Urology, Humanitas Clinical and Research Institute, Rozzano, Italy

2 Humanitas University, Pieve Emanuele, Italy

*Address all correspondence to: buffi.nicolomaria@gmail.com


IntechOpen

## References

[1] Schuessler WW, Grune MT, Tecuanhuey LV, et al. Laparoscopic dismembered pyeloplasty. The Journal of Urology. 1993;**150**:1795

[2] Brooks JD, Kavoussi LR, Preminger GM, Schessler WW. Comparison of open and endourological approaches to the obstructed uretero-pelvic junction. Urology. 1995;**46**:791-795

[3] Bauer JJ, Bishoff JT, Moore RG, Chen RN, Iverson AJ, Kavoussi LR. Laparoscopic versus open pyeloplasty: Assessment of objective and subjective out-come. The Journal of Urology. 1999;**162**:692-695

[4] Klingler HC, Remzi M, Janetschek G, Kratzik C, Marberger MJ. Comparison of open versus laparoscopic pyeloplasty techniques in treatment of ureteropelvic junction obstruction. European Urology. 2003;**44**:340-345

[5] Cestari A, Buffi NM, Lista G, et al. Retroperitoneal and transperitoneal robot-assisted pyeloplasty in adults: Techniques and results. European Urology. 2010;**58**:711-718

[6] Gettman MT, Neururer R, Bartsch G, Peschel R. Anderson-Hynes dismembered pyeloplasty performed using the da Vinci robotic system. Urology. 2002;**60**:509-513

[7] Cestari A, Guazzoni G, Naspro R, et al. Original dissecting balloon for retroperitoneal laparoscopy: Cost-effective alternative to commercially available device. Journal of Endourology. 2007;**21**:714-717

[8] Gupta NP, Mukherjee S, Nayyar R, Hemal AK, Kumar R. Transmesocolic robot-assisted pyeloplasty: Single center experience. Journal of Endourology. 2009;**23**:945-948

[9] Porpiglia F, Billia M, Volpe A, Morra I, Scarpa RM. Transperitoneal left laparoscopic pyeloplasty with transmesocolic access to the pelvi-ureteric junction: Technique description and results with a minimum follow-up of 1 year. BJU International. 2008;**101**:1024-1028

[10] Shadpour P, Nayyeri RK, Daneshvar R, Salimi H, Radfar H. Prospective clinical trial to compare standard colon-reflecting with transmesocolic laparoscopic pyeloplasty. BJU International. 2012;**110**:1814-1818

[11] Minervini A, Siena G, Masieri L, Lapini A, Serni S, Carini M. Antegrade stenting in laparoscopic pyeloplasty: Feasibility of the technique and time required for stent insertion. Surgical Endoscopy. 2009;**23**:1831-1834

[12] Rodrigues H, Rodrigues P, Ruela M, Bernabé A, Buogo G. Dismembered laparoscopic pyeloplasty with antegrade placement of ureteral stent: Simplification of the technique. International Brazilian Journal of Urology. 2002;**28**:439-444

[13] Gaitonde K, Roesel G, Donovan J. Novel technique of retrograde ureteral stenting during laparoscopic pyeloplasty. Journal of Endourology. 2008;**22**:1199-1202

[14] Fiori C, Morra I, Di Stasio A, Grande S, Scarpa RM, Porpiglia F. Flexible pneumocystoscopy for double J stenting during laparoscopic and robot assisted pyeloplasty: Our experience. International Journal of Urology. 2010;**17**:192-194

[15] Mandhani A, Goel S, Bhandari M. Is antegrade stenting superior to retrograde stenting in laparoscopic pyeloplasty? The Journal of Urology. 2004;**171**:1440-1442

[16] Chandrasekharam VV. Is retrograde stenting more reliable than antegrade stenting for pyeloplasty in infants and children? Urology. 2005;**66**:1301-1304

[17] Arumainayagam N, Minervini A, Davenport K, et al. Antegrade versus retrograde stenting in laparoscopic pyeloplasty. Journal of Endourology. 2008;**22**:671-674

[18] El-Feel AS, Abdel-Hakim MA, Abouel-Fettouh HI, Abdel-Hakim AM. Antegrade ureteral stenting during laparoscopic dismembered pyeloplasty: Intraoperative findings and long-term outcome. Journal of Endourology. 2010;**24**:551-555

[19] Shalhav AL, Mikhail AA, Orvieto MA, Gofrit ON, Gerber GS, Zorn KC. Adult stentless laparoscopic pyeloplasty. Journal of the Society of Laparoendoscopic Surgeons. 2007;**11**:8-13

[20] Bilen CY, Bayazit Y, Güdelo lu A, Abat D, Inci K, Doran S. Laparoscopic pyeloplasty in adults: Stented versus stentless. Journal of Endourology. 2011;**25**:645-650

[21] Sethi AS, Regan SM, Sundaram CP. Robot-assisted laparoscopic pyeloplasty with and without a ureteral stent. Journal of Endourology. 2011;**25**:239-243

[22] Patel V. Robotic-assisted laparoscopic dismembered pyeloplasty. Urology. 2005;**66**:45-49

[23] Mufarrij PW, Woods M, Shah OD, et al. Robotic dismembered pyeloplasty: A 6-year, multi- institutional experience. The Journal of Urology. 2008;**180**:1391-1396

[24] Schwentner C, Pelzer A, Neururer R, et al. Robotic Anderson-Hynes pyeloplasty: 5-year experience of one Centre. BJU International. 2007;**100**:880-885

[25] Sivaraman A, Leveillee RJ, Patel MB, et al. Robot- assisted laparoscopic dismembered pyeloplasty for ureteropelvic junction obstruction: A multi-institutional experience. Urology. 2012;**79**:351-355

[26] Gupta NP, Nayyar R, Hemal AK, Mukherjee S, Kumar R, Dogra PN. Outcome analysis of robotic pyeloplasty: A large single-Centre experience. BJU International. 2010;**105**:980-983

[27] Autorino R, Eden C, El-Ghoneimi A, et al. Robot-assisted and laparoscopic repair of ureteropelvic junction obstruction: A systematic review and metanalysis. European Urology. 2014;**65**:430-452

[28] Minnillo BJ, Cruz JA, Sayao RH, et al. Long-term experience and outcomes of robotic assisted laparoscopic pyeloplasty in children and young adults. The Journal of Urology. 2011;**185**:1455-1460

[29] Cundy TP, Harling L, Hughes-Hallett A, et al. Meta-analysis of robot-assisted vs conventional laparoscopic and open pyeloplasty in children: Robot- assisted vs laparoscopic and open pyeloplasty in children. BJU International. 2014;**114**:582-594

[30] Olsen LH, Rawashdeh YF, Jorgensen TM. Pediatric robot assisted retroperitoneoscopic pyeloplasty: A 5-year experience. Journal of Urology. 2007;**178**(5):2137-2141

[31] Gupta NP, Nayyar R, Hemal AK, et al. Outcome analysis of robotic pyeloplasty: A large single-centre experience. BJU International. 2010;**105**(7):980-983. DOI: 10.1111/j.1464-410X.2009.08983

[32] Etafy M, Pick D, Said S, et al. Robotic pyeloplasty: The University of California-Irvine experience. Journal of Urology. 2011;**185**(6):2196-2200. DOI: 10.1016/j.juro.2011.02.054

[33] Buffi NM, Lughezzani G, Hurle R, et al. Robot-assisted surgery for benign ureteral strictures: Experience and outcomes from four tertiary care institutions. European Urology. 2017;**71**:945-951

[34] Dangle PP, Akhavan A, Odeleye M, et al. Ninety-day perioperative complications of pediatric robotic urological surgery: A multi-institutional study. Journal of Pediatric Urology. 2016;**12**(102):e1-e102

[35] Basatac C, Boylu U, Öno FF, Gümüs E. Comparison of surgical and functional outcomes of open, laparoscopic and robotic pyeloplasty for the treatment of ureteropelvic junction obstruction. Turkish Journal of Urology. 2014;**40**(1):24-30

[36] Hanske J, Sanchez A, et al. Comparison of 30-day perioperative outcomes in adults undergoing open versus minimally invasive pyeloplasty for uretero-pelvic junction obstruction: Analysis of 593 patients in a prospective national database. World Journal of Urology. 2015;**33**(12):2107-2113

[37] Mei H, Pu J, Yang C, Zhang H, Zheng L, Tong Q. Laparoscopic versus open pyeloplasty for ureteropelvic junction obstruction in children: A systematic review and meta-analysis. Journal of Endourology. 2011;**25**:727-736

[38] Thom MR, Haseebuddin M, Roytman TM, Benway BM, Bhayani SB, FigenshauRS. Robot-assistedpyeloplasty: Outcomes for primary and secondary repairs, a single institution experience. International Braz J Urol. 2012;**38**:77-83

[39] Atug F, Burgess SV, Castle EP, Thomas R. Role of robotics in the management of secondary ureteropelvic junction obstruction. International Journal of Clinical Practice. 2006;**60**:9-11

[40] Hemal AK, Mishra S, Mukharjee S, Suryavanshi M. Robot assisted laparoscopic pyeloplasty in patients of ureteropelvic junction obstruction with previously failed open surgical repair. International Journal of Urology. 2008;**15**:744-746

[41] Lindgren BW, Hagerty J, Meyer T, Cheng EY. Robot- assisted laparoscopic reoperative repair for failed pyeloplasty in children: A safe and highly effective treatment option. The Journal of Urology. 2012;**188**:932-937

[42] Niver BE, Agalliu I, Bareket R, Mufarrij P, Shah O, Stifelman MD. Analysis of robotic-assisted laparoscopic pyeloplasty for primary versus secondary repair in 119 consecutive cases. Urology. 2012;**79**:689-694

[43] Desai MM, Berger AK, Brandina R, et al. Laparoendoscopic single-site surgery: Initial hundred patients. Urology. 2009;**74**:805-812

[44] White WM, Haber GP, Goel RK, Crouzet S, Stein RJ, Kaouk JH. Single port urologic surgery: Single center experience with the first 100 cases. Urology. 2009;**74**:801-804

[45] Cestari A, Buffi NM, Lista G, et al. Feasibility and preliminary clinical outcomes of robotic laparoendoscopic single-site (R-LESS) pyeloplasty using a new single-port platform. European Urology. 2012;**62**(1):175-179

[46] Buffi NM, Lughezzani G, Fossati N, et al. Robot-assisted, single-site, dismembered pyeloplasty for ureteropelvic junction obstruction with the new da Vinci platform: A stage 2a study. European Urology. 2015;**67**:151-156

[47] Zhao LC, Weinberg AC, Lee Z, et al. Robotic ureteral reconstruction using buccal mucosa grafts: A multi-institutional experience. European Urology. 2018;**73**:419-426

[48] Ahn JJ, Shapiro ME, Ellison JS, et al. Pediatric robot-assisted redo pyeloplasty with buccal mucosa graft: A novel technique. Urology. 2017;**101**:56-59

[49] Zampini AM, Nelson R, Haijing Zhang JJ, et al. Robotic salvage pyeloplasty with buccal mucosal onlay graft: Video demonstration of technique and outcomes. Urology. 2017;**110**:253-256

[50] Lee Z, Moore B, Giusto L, Eun DD. Use of indocyanine green during robot-assisted ureteral reconstructions. European Urology. 2015;**67**:291-298

[51] Diana P, Lughezzani G, Maffei D, et al. Intraureteral indocyanine green in robot-assisted re-do pyeloplasty for recurrent ureteropelvic junction obstruction. European Urology Supplements. 2019;**18**:e2730. DOI: 10.1016/S1569-9056(19)32827-1

[52] Cinman NM, Okeke Z, Smith ADJ. Pelvic kidney: Associated diseases and treatment. Endourology. 2007;**21**:836-842

Chapter 7

# Robotic-Assisted Inguinal Lymphadenectomy (RAIL)

*Victor Enrique Corona-Montes, Eduardo Gonzalez-Cuenca and Marcos Tobias-Machado*

## Abstract

The objective of the following chapter is to describe thoroughly the surgical technique for a robotic-assisted inguinal lymphadenectomy for penile cancer, and the surgery has been through modifications from its creation to "the Robotic Era." Penile cancer is a rare neoplasm, with an estimated 1570 cases in the United States. The spread is predictable to the inguinal lymph nodes, where 1–2% of patients will present distant metastases. The first draining lymph area is found in the inguinal region and the secondary spread in the pelvic region, main reason for the inguinal part of the treatment of penile cancer under different indications. Radical resection of inguinal metastases of penile cancer is the standard treatment for this technique, which has been adapted to become a minimally invasive surgery compared to an open inguinal lymphadenectomy, which entails a high incidence of morbidity that stands at 50–90%. A robotic-assisted inguinal lymphadenectomy, despite its high cost, is a feasible technique when carried out in specialized centers that can reduce morbidity rates and offer good oncological results, less blood loss, and shorter hospital stay.

**Keywords:** inguinal dissection, penile cancer, robotic surgery

## 1. Introduction

In 2002, Ian M. Thompson and Jay T. Bishop conceived the idea of an endoscopic and subcutaneous approach for inguinal lymph node dissection applying laparoscopic techniques. The endoscopic subcutaneous approach for a modified inguinal lymphadenectomy (ESMIL) procedure was described in a cadaveric model and performed in 2003 on a patient with T3N1M0 squamous cell carcinoma of the penis with an adequate identification of anatomical landmarks and overall feasibility [1]. In 2007, Tobias-Machado et al. reported reduced complications (20% vs 70%), shorter hospitalization times, more favorable cosmetic outcomes, and optimal oncologic outcomes regarding a refined technique coined as "video-endoscopic inguinal lymphadenectomy" (VEIL), in contrast with more traditional open procedures [2, 3].

International literature proclaimed the benefits and fewer complications that minimally invasive lymph node resection implied, such as skin necrosis without compromising oncologic control. These facts paved the way for new technological advances to be employed, as in the case for the "robotic-assisted inguinal lymphadenectomy" (RAIL). This robotic technology allows for a three-dimensional operative field, tremor filter, and articulated instruments, which grant the surgeon improved visibility, identification of anatomical landmarks, dexterity, and improved ergonomics, thus overcoming the limitations of VEIL. Josephson and associates were the first to describe the feasibility of a nonsimultaneous bilateral RAIL using the da Vinci S robotic system [4].

In 2013, Matin et al. published a prospective study where the oncologic efficacy of RAIL to adequately stage the disease was confirmed, with an independent surgeon assessment by a direct visual evaluation of the dissection field through a small inguinal incision [5]. Russell also described a lower complication rate of the RAIL approach in comparison with VEIL technique (10% vs. 40%), although the group of VEIL patients was smaller [6]. Sotelo et al. and Ahlawat et al. have described different techniques that allows for a simultaneous bilateral RAIL to be performed without moving the robotic system across the operating room and maintaining an adequate reproducibility as well as allowing a bilateral staging procedure in the same surgical time [7, 8].

The author of the chapter described the first RAIL carried out in Mexico in the year 2015. It was performed on a 73-year-old patient with squamous cell carcinoma of the penis (T3N0M0G1), and he underwent a radical penectomy 4 weeks earlier the lymphadenectomy. The bilateral RAIL using the da Vinci Si HD surgical system was performed, and both saphenous veins were successfully preserved [9].

New technological advances, refinements, and modifications in the minimally invasive lymph node dissection technique will continue to reduce the morbidity and complications and improve the quality of life of the penile cancer patient.

## 2. Epidemiology of penile cancer

Penile cancer is a rare neoplasm, making up for less than an estimated 1% of all types of cancer in the United States, translating to an approximate amount of 2100 new cases and 400 deaths annually [9]. According to the Global Cancer Observatory, the estimated number of incident cases is 34,475 and a mortality of 15,138 cases in all ages [10]. This type of cancer is more common in less developed areas of the world (i.e., Africa, Asia, and South America), where it accounts up to 10–20% of all malignancies in men. Penile cancer is considered a disease that typically affects older men, where males between ages 55 and 58 are more prone to be affected.

This tumor is unusual in younger patients (<40 years old), although cases have been reported [11]. The ethnicity has been demonstrated to have no impact in the incidence, but it does play a role as a risk factor regarding survival outcomes (it is worse for African-American ethnicities).

Multiple factors are associated with a risk of developing penile cancer, such as suffering from genital warts (OR 7.6), penile tears (OR 5.2), chronic penile rash (OR 3.2), penile injuries (OR 3.5), phimosis (seven times higher risk), human papilloma virus (DNA identified >30%), human immunodeficiency virus (4–8 times higher risk), tobacco exposure (3 times more likely), and lichen sclerosis (balanitis xerotica obliterans) [12].

The spread is predictable to the inguinal lymph nodes, where only 1–2% of patients will present distant metastases. Approximately 20% of patients with clinically nonpalpable inguinal nodes harbor occult metastases. The first draining lymph node group is found both in the superficial and in the deep inguinal region (superomedial zone), whereas the second lymph node group spread lies in the ipsilateral pelvic region and, lastly, in the retroperitoneum (para-caval/para-aortic lymph nodes) [13].

Penile cancer patients in the low-risk group (Tis, Ta, T1G1, No LVI) have a <16% metastatic rate to the lymph nodes, intermediate risk (T1G2) have 17–50%, and high risk (T1G3, >T2, LVI) have 68–73% metastatic rate [14].

Radical resection of inguinal metastases of penile cancer is the standard treatment, and the greatest single predictor of survival in squamous cell carcinoma of the penis is the incidence and extent of lymph node involvement [11, 14]. The objective of the lymph node resection is providing accurate pathology staging and if disease exists in the nodes alter its natural history and pattern of metastasis. Men found to have a single node involved (N1) had a 100% 3-year disease-specific survival. The presence of 1–3 involved nodes predicts a 5-year overall survival rate of 75.6%, whereas for 4 or 5 nodes involved the rate is at 8.4 and 0% for patients with more than 5 positive nodes [14].

This technique has been adapted as a minimally invasive surgery, and in comparison with the open inguinal lymphadenectomy, it preferred because of the latter's high incidence of morbidity that stands a 50–90% rate regarding an open approach [2]. Robotic-assisted inguinal lymphadenectomy, aside from its high cost, is a feasible technique when carried out in specialized centers reduces morbidity and provides adequate oncological results, less blood loss, and shorter hospital stay.

## 3. Anatomical aspects

The femoral vessels are found in the femoral triangle and formed laterally by the sartorius muscle laterally, superiorly by the inguinal ligament superiorly, and medially by the long adductor medially. The junction between the saphenous and femoral vessels is located approximately two fingerbreadths lateral and two fingerbreadths inferior to the pubic tubercle. The saphenous vein passes anteriorly through the fossa ovalis and elapses with the superficial inguinal region. The structures that will be found in the femoral triangle are (from lateral to medial) femoral nerve, the femoral artery, the femoral vein, and the deep inguinal lymph nodes. These last three are located inside the femoral sheath [13] **Figure 1**.

The fascia lata separates the inguinal lymph nodes into superficial and deep groups. The superficial inguinal lymph nodes are situated in the deep membranous layer of the superficial fascia of the thigh (Camper's fascia), approximately composed by 4 or up to 25 nodes. The superficial inguinal nodes have been divided into 5 anatomic groups by Daseler in 1948 [13, 15] (**Figure 2**).

1. Superomedial nodes (I) around the superficial external pudendal and superficial epigastric veins.

2. Superolateral nodes (II) around the superficial circumflex vein.

3. Inferolateral nodes (III) around the lateral femoral cutaneous and superficial circumflex veins.

4. Inferomedial nodes (IV) around the greater saphenous vein.

5. Central nodes (V) around the saphenofemoral junction.

The superficial external pudendal vein, superficial circumflex vein, and the lateral femoral cutaneous vein are branches of the greater saphenous vein (**Figure 3**).

The deep inguinal nodes are located deep into the fascia lata and lie medial to the femoral vein in the femoral triangle. The node of Cloquet is the most cephalad node in the deep inguinal region, located between the femoral vein and the lacunar ligament.

The standard or full template for the inguinal lymph node dissection includes Daseler's 5 group nodes in the superficial dissection and the deep

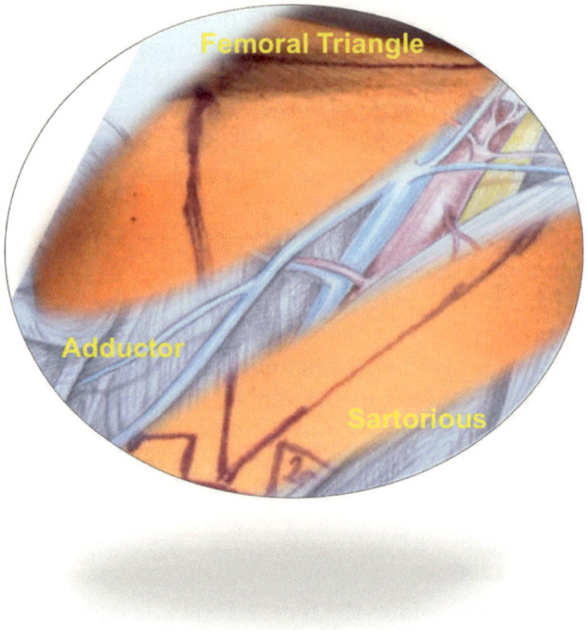


**Figure 1.**
*Femoral triangle (left limb).*

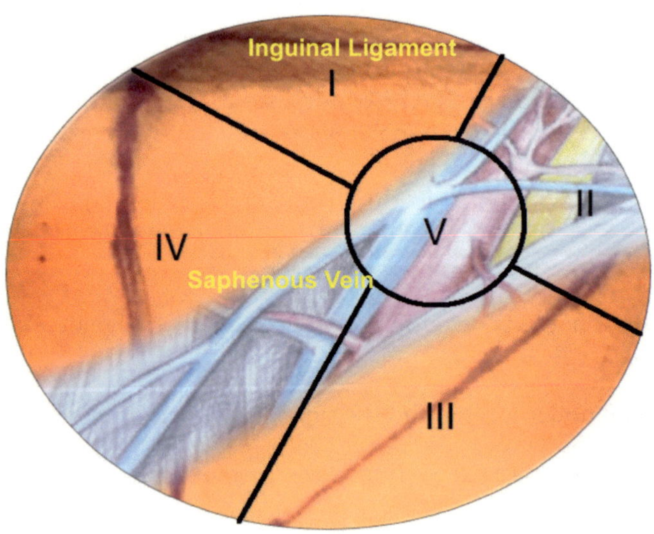


**Figure 2.**
*Schematics of Daseler zones (left limb).*

inguinal nodes from the femoral triangle, limiting the dissection lateral to the femoral artery, which eliminates the risk of injury to the femoral nerve. This template includes the ligation of the saphenous vein as it emerges from the femoral vein. The template requires the superficial dissection of the first group lymph nodes entirely, as well as a portion of the second and fifth group lymph nodes, the inferior group nodes are not dissected, the deep dissection remains the same. The modified template was described to reduce the complication rate, which can be also accomplished by the minimally invasive approach.

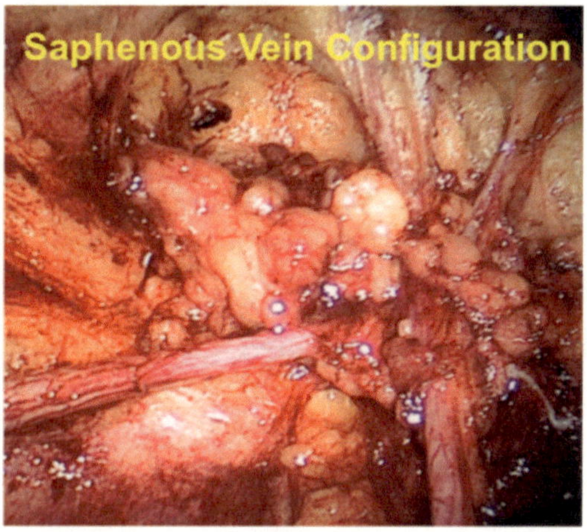


**Figure 3.**
*Saphenous vein configuration.*

## 4. Surgical indications for RAIL

The treatment of regional lymph nodes is decisive for patient survival. A cure for the disease confined to regional nodes can be achieved and a radical lymphadenectomy is the treatment of choice. For this section, a description of the actual surgical indications for inguinal lymphadenectomy in the different group risks and clinical stages will be presented [16, 17].

### 4.1 Patients with clinically normal inguinal lymph nodes (cN0)

Micrometastatic disease occurs in up to 25% of the patients and invasive lymph node staging is necessary. The indication for an inguinal lymphadenectomy is for intermediate (T1b, Grade 1 or 2) and high-risk tumors (T1b, Grade 3 or 4; any T2 or greater), which are considered to have an elevated risk of lymphatic spread. The superficial inguinal lymphadenectomy is an option that can be completed (radical) if one pathological lymph node is found without extranodal extension. If extranodal extension is present or ≥2 lymph nodes are positive, inguinal and pelvic lymphadenectomy should be considered.

### 4.2 Patients with palpable uni- or bilateral inguinal nodes (cN1/cN2)

Metastatic disease is very likely and lymph node surgery (radical inguinal lymphadenectomy) with histopathology is necessary. Treatment in these patients should not be delayed given that the metastatic spread continues. If a high-risk primary lesion was identified, a complete inguinal lymphadenectomy + contralateral superficial lymphadenectomy should be performed. If ≥2 inguinal nodes are positive or ≥1 inguinal node is positive with extranodal extension, an ipsilateral pelvic lymph node dissection is recommended to be performed.

### 4.3 Patients with bulky inguinal nodes

In this scenario, the patients will require multimodal treatment consisting of chemotherapy and surgery. The radical inguinal lymphadenectomy will be indicated after a positive metastatic (fine needle aspiration) disease in unilateral mobile ≥4 cm lymph node. If ≥2 nodes are positive or have extranodal extension, a pelvic lymphadenectomy should be performed and adjuvant chemotherapy considered. In the scenario where the lymph node is ≥4 cm and fixed or mobile bilateral, neoadjuvant chemotherapy should be administrated after the positive finding in the fine needle aspiration, followed by inguinal and pelvic lymphadenectomy if an adequate response to chemotherapy was documented.

In others of RAIL, descriptions the patients staging where up to cN2 and less than 3 cm in size lymph nodes, as equal for VEIL studies (**Figure 4**).

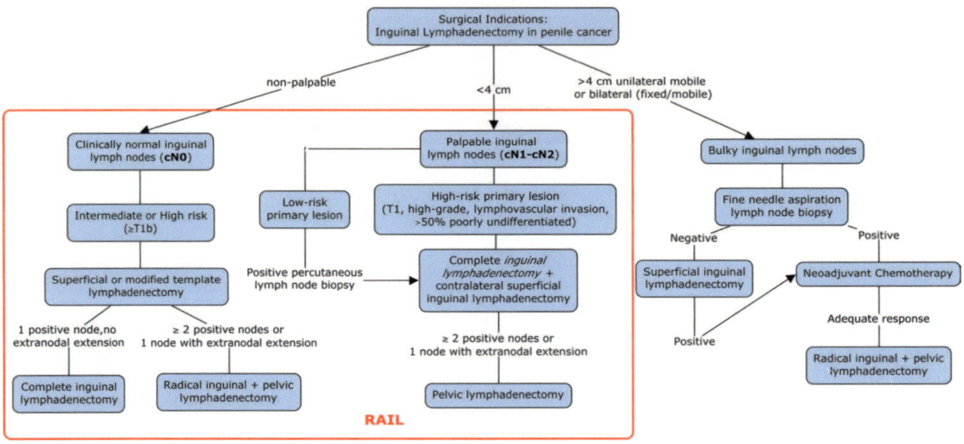


**Figure 4.**
*Surgical indications for inguinal lymphadenectomy in penile cancer.*

### 4.4 Patient preparation and position

An initial challenge presents itself at the beginning of the procedure: the positioning of the da Vinci robot and the operation table. Initially, the robot was placed on the right side of the table, considering it was an SI system that did not require repositioning but simply redocking of the instruments. As a first step, the operating field is prepared and readied by having the patients lie in the dorsal decubitus position with abduction of both legs dressed since the beginning of the procedure to avoid time loss.

The preparation is then followed by realizing a medial incision localized in the femoral triangle, inside the Sartorius muscle and joint with the adductor longus. A 3 cm incision is realized 5 cm over the knee, under protection of the skin and small fatty tissue from the leg, we follow a digital dissection in direction of the inguinal ligament. This blunt finger dissection is accompanied with movements to the left and right sides of the thigh and heading also as upper as possible. The previous dissection is realized for the superficial plane of the lymph's (**Figure 5**).

### 4.5 Surgical technique

#### *4.5.1 Trocar placement: anterior, lateral, and posterior boundaries*

Once we have created this space manually, three more incisions will be performed. The first, a 5 mm one that will serve as a laparoscopic port, is placed 2 cm medial and below the initial incision of the left leg, while replicating this incision on the right leg (on its lateral side) and at the same distance, also 2 cm, so that the assistant port is external to the position of both legs. Right away, one of the robotic ports is placed 2 cm higher on the external side of the left leg, and one more robotic

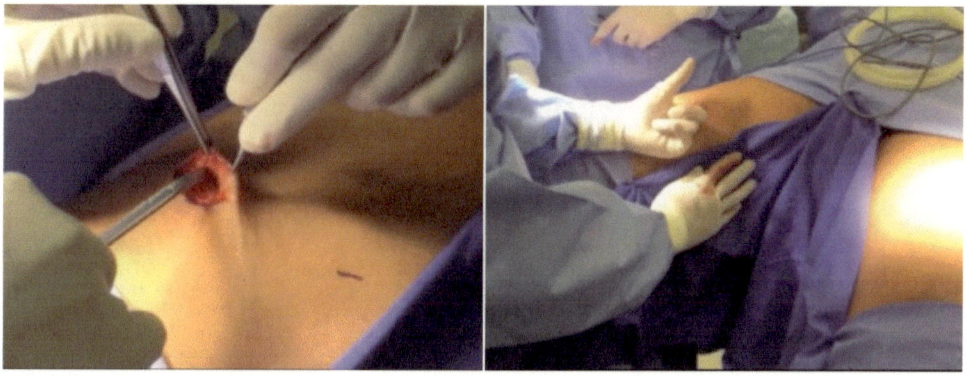

**Figure 5.**
*Skin incision and finger dissection.*

port is situated 3 cm to the left of the initial incision, on the same leg. This is where the camera port will be placed.

For the right leg, the first robotic port is placed 2 cm higher on the leg's external side, and the second robotic port is located 3 cm to the right of the initial incision on this leg. This description is done simultaneously so that both legs are ready to dock the robot.

In the case of da Vinci X or Xi, right-side placement is also performed simply with a redocking of the arms, which allow for smaller incisions and for the camera to be changed to another robotic port, as well as the advantage of an easier, faster, and better position in the middle of the abducted legs of the patient. For every kind of model of the da Vinci systems, we use 0° lens, and once the ports are installed, the $CO_2$ insufflation is managed at 10 mmHg (**Figure 6**).

Once the docking is done, under the da Vinci system's 0° lens, the anatomical references of the femoral triangle and the packet of superficial nodes are located over the fascia lata. When performing a deep node dissection, we transected the fascia lata with each trocar staying laterally to the adductor longus and sartorius muscles doing a work below the fascia. The $CO_2$ insufflation creates a working space, so we follow the middle of the muscles to find femoral nerve and vessels removing the femoral nodes (**Figure 7**).

After this, the trocars are slightly pulled up (without redocking) hence staying only on the superficial level. We lift up the superficial packet and follow the packet to the inguinal ligament, lateral to the saphenous vein, which is not always respect but transected, going higher to the saphenofemoral junction, an reaching the superficial nodes packet **Figure 8.**

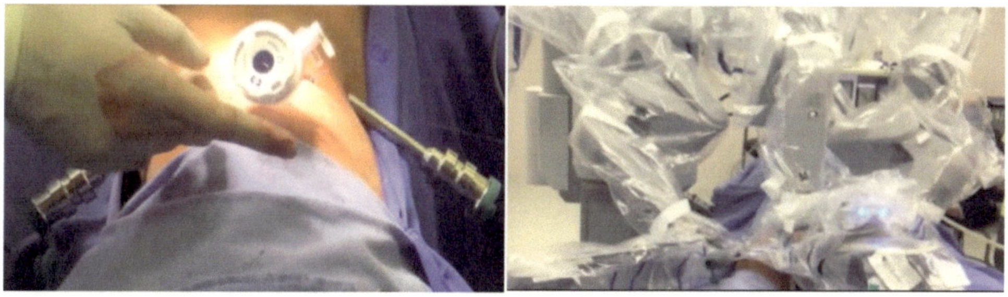

**Figure 6.**
*Trocars' position and docking.*

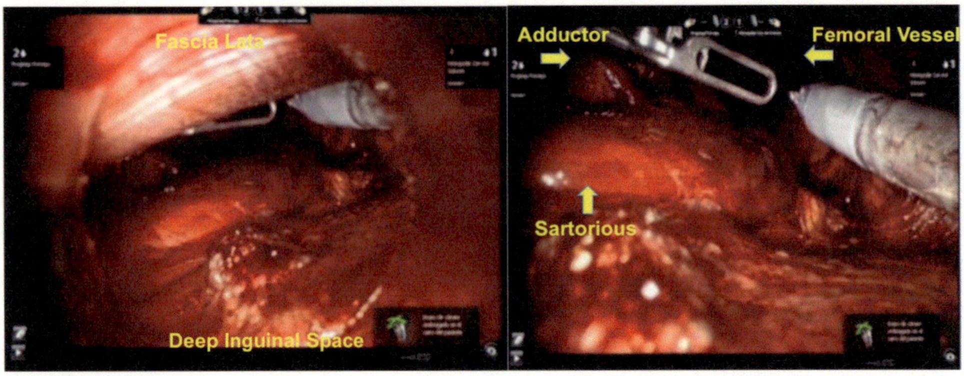


**Figure 7.**
*Deep inguinal space.*

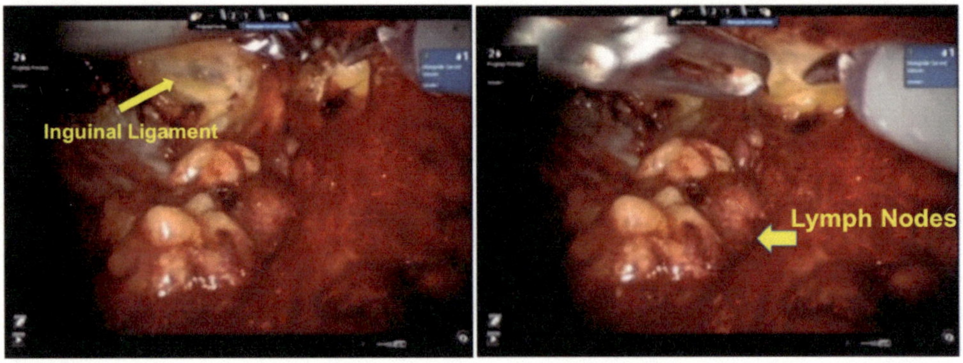


**Figure 8.**
*Inguinal ligament and superficial nodes.*

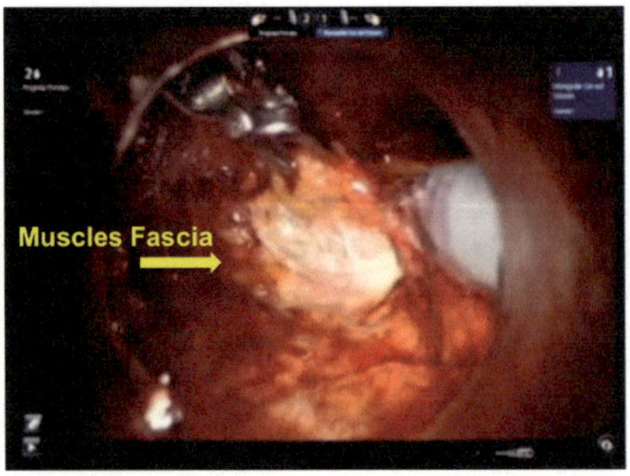


**Figure 9.**
*Muscles fascia.*

The control of the saphenofemoral junction can be performed with either metallic clips or 10 mm hem-o-lok; this junction is found over the muscles fascia in the interior side of the leg (**Figure 9**).

The packet is placed in an endobag and removed via the initial incision or the camera's main port. A drain is placed in each leg through the 5-mm incision trocar. See **Figure 10**.

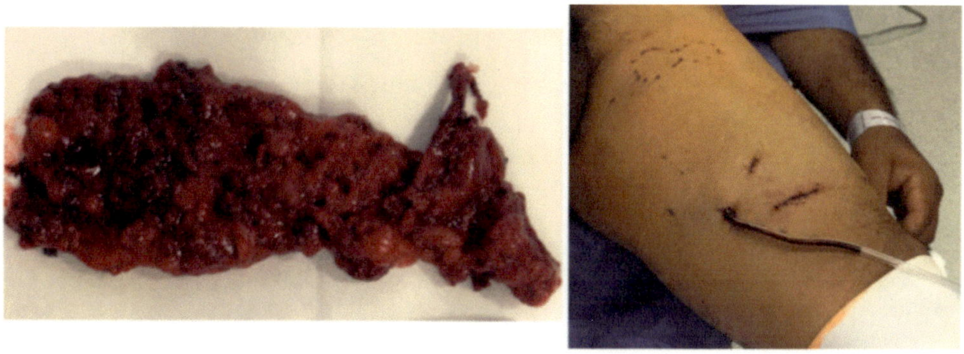

**Figure 10.**
*Nodes packet and drain.*

## 5. Our experience

Between 2015 and 2018, we have performed 12 cases (24 limbs) of robotic inguinal lymph node dissection, where the patient's median age was 58 years old. A 100% of the patients had been diagnosed with penile squamous cell carcinoma, confirmed by biopsy, and had previously experienced a partial or total penectomy. The TNM for the patients was T2–3, cN1–2, M0, G1–3. Operative room mean time was 110 min (range 90–230 min). The mean blood loss was 59 ml (35–85). None of the surgeries were converted to an open approach. The total mean number of dissected lymph was 148 and mean lymph nodes per case were 12, and from those, 1.8 were positive for SCC per limb (n = 22 positive lymph nodes). Hospitalization median stay was 2.5 days (range 2–4 days), and the duration of the drainage on overage 16 days (range 10–21 days). Complications were classified as Clavien-Dindo III (lymphocele: 2/24) whom needed single percutaneous drainage and 10 days of antibiotic treatment, however, did not require any hospital stay (**Tables 1** and **2**).

| | |
|---|---|
| No. of patients (limbs) | 12 (24) |
| Age (range) | 58 years old (41–73) |
| Histological type | Penile SCC |
| Operative time (range) | 110 min (90–230) |
| Blood loss (range) | 59 ml (35–85) |
| Conversion to open surgery | None |
| Total of dissected lymph nodes (mean per patient) | 148 (12) |
| No. of total positive nodes (mean per patient) | 22 (1.8) |
| Hospital stay (range) | 2.5 days (2–4) |
| Duration of drainage (range) | 16 days (10–21) |
| Postoperative complications (n) | Lymphocele (2/12) |

**Table 1.**
*Description group.*

| Author | Year | Case report/ case series | Number of patients (# limbs) | Age (mean -years) | Penile cancer (histologic) | T stage | Pre-LND cN stage | Lymph nodes dissected (n) - mean | Operative time (min) | Blood loss (mL) | Complications |
|---|---|---|---|---|---|---|---|---|---|---|---|
| Josephson et al. [4] | 2009 | Case report | 1 (2) | 37 | SCC◆ | T3 | cN2 | 10/9* | 120/130* | 100/50* | None |
| Matin et al. [5] | 2013 | Case series | 10 (20) | 62 | SCC◆ | T1–3 | cN0-cN1 | Left: 9, Right: 9 | 180–240 | 100 (mean) | Cellulitis (2/10), wound breakdown (2/10), skin necrosis (1/10) |
| Sotelo et al. [6] | 2013 | Case report | 1 (2) | 64 | SCC◆ | T3 | cN0 | 33 | 360 | 100 | Lymphocele |
| Corona-Montes et al. [9] | 2015 | Case report | 1 (2) | 73 | SCC◆ | T3 | cN0 | NA | 230 | 50 | None |
| Ahlawat et al. [7] | 2016 | Case series | 3 (6) | 56 | SCC◆ | T2-T3 | cN1-cN2 | Left: 18, Right: 14 | 453 | 147 (mean) | Lymphocele (1/3) |
| Our experience | 2018 | Case series | 12 (24) | 58 | SCC◆ | T2-T3 | cN1-cN2 | 12 | 110 | 59 (mean) | Lymphocele (2/12) |

**RAIL performed in two separate procedures (one OR time per limb).*
*◆Squamous cell carcinoma of the penis.*

**Table 2.**
*RAIL comparative reports.*

## 6. Conclusions

The robotic inguinal lymphadenectomy for penile cancer is still a novel technique that requires further studies to thoroughly demonstrate its utility. The open approach has shown an increased morbidity and rate of complications, primary producing flap skin necrosis, longer hospitalization stays, and infections. On the contrary, RAIL provides a three-dimensional vision and improved dexterity thanks to the articulated instruments that allow surgeons to work in a very reduced workspace, produce less surgical trauma to the skin, reduce operative time (while winning experience in anatomy field and in the docking of the robot), and perform both superficial and deep lymphadenectomy in both legs as previous approaches. The challenges for the aforementioned robotic approach are not only the high costs implied but also the learning curve for the femoral triangle anatomy and anatomical variations. There is not enough prospective evidence about robotic inguinal approach for penile cancer, but what can be affirmed is that the previously presented evidence report not only less morbidity with minimally invasive techniques (VEIL, RAIL) and equal oncologic results.

## Conflict of interest

The authors declare no conflict of interest.

## Notes/Thanks/Other declarations

Thanks to collaborative group.

## Nomenclature

| | |
|---|---|
| ESMIL | endoscopic subcutaneous modified inguinal lymphadenectomy |
| VEIL | video-endoscopic inguinal lymphadenectomy |
| RAIL | robotic-assisted inguinal lymphadenectomy |

## Author details

Victor Enrique Corona-Montes[1*], Eduardo Gonzalez-Cuenca[2] and Marcos Tobias-Machado[3]

1 General Hospital of México/American British Cowdray Hospital (A.B.C), México City, Mexico

2 General Hospital of México, México City, Mexico

3 Department of Urology, Medicine School of ABC, Sao Paulo, Brazil

*Address all correspondence to: urocorona@hotmail.com

## References

[1] Bishoff JT, Lackland AFB, Basler JW, Teichman JM, Thompson IM. Endoscopic subcutaneous modified inguinal lymph node dissection (ESMIL) for squamous cell carcinoma of the penis. Journal of Urology. 2003;**169**(suppl):78. abstract 301

[2] Tobias-Machado M, Tavares A, Ornellas AA, Molina WR, Juliano RV, Wroclawski ER. Video endoscopic inguinal lymphadenectomy: A new minimally invasive procedure for radical management of inguinal nodes in patients with penile squamous cell carcinoma. Juro. 2007;**177**:953-7–discussion958. DOI: 10.1016/j.juro.2006.10.075

[3] Tobias-Machado M, Tavares A, Silva MNR, Molina WR, Forseto PH, Juliano RV, et al. Can video endoscopic inguinal lymphadenectomy achieve a lower morbidity than open lymph node dissection in penile cancer patients? Journal of Endourology. 2008;**22**:1687-1691. DOI: 10.1089/end.2007.0386

[4] Josephson DY, Jacobsohn KM, Link BA, Wilson TG. Robotic-assisted endoscopic inguinal lymphadenectomy. 2009;73:167-170. doi:10.1016/j.urology.2008.05.060

[5] Matin SF, Cormier JN, Ward JF, Pisters LL, Wood CG, Dinney CPN, et al. Phase 1 prospective evaluation of the oncological adequacy of robotic assisted video-endoscopic inguinal lymphadenectomy in patients with penile carcinoma. BJU International. 2013;**111**:1068-1074. DOI: 10.1111/j.1464-410X.2012.11729.x

[6] Sotelo R, Cabrera M, Carmona O, de Andrade R, Martin O, Fernandez G. Robotic bilateral inguinal lymphadenectomy in penile cancer, development of a technique without robot repositioning: A case report. Ecancermedicalscience. 2013;7:356. DOI: 10.3332/ecancer.2013.356

[7] Ahlawat R, Khera R, Gautam G, Kumar A. Robot-assisted simultaneous bilateral radical inguinal lymphadenectomy along with robotic bilateral pelvic lymphadenectomy: A feasibility study. Journal of Laparoendoscopic & Advanced Surgical Techniques. Part A. 2016;**26**:845-849. DOI: 10.1089/lap.2015.0611

[8] Siegel RL, Miller KD, Jemal A. Cancer statistics, 2019. CA: A Cancer Journal for Clinicians. 2019;**69**:7-34. DOI: 10.3322/caac.21551

[9] Corona-Montes VE, Moyo-Martínez E, Almazán-Treviño L, Ríos-Dávila V, Santiago-Hernández Y, Mendoza-Rojas EE. Linfadenectomía inguinal robot asistida (LIRA) para cáncer de pene. Revista Mexicana de Urología. 2015;**75**:292-296. DOI: 10.1016/j.uromx.2015.06.006

[10] Global Cancer Observatory. Cancer Today [Internet]. 2018. Available from: https://gco.iarc.fr

[11] Pettaway CA, Crook J, Pagliaro L. Tumor of the penis. In: Wein A, Kavoussi L, Partin A, editors. Campbell-Walsh Urology. 11th ed. Philadelphia: Elsevier; 2016. pp. 846-878

[12] Daling JR, Madeleine MM, Johnson LG, Schwartz SM, Shera KA, Wurscher MA, et al. Penile cancer: Importance of circumcision, human papillomavirus and smoking in in situ and invasive disease. International Journal of Cancer. 2005;**116**:606-616. DOI: 10.1002/ijc.21009

[13] Angermeier K, Sotelo R, Sharp D. Inguinal node dissection. In: Wein A, Kavoussi L, Partin A, editors. Campbell-Walsh Urology. 11th ed. Philadelphia: Elsevier; 2016. pp. 846-878

[14] Hegarty PK, Dinney CP, Pettaway CA. Controversies in ilioinguinal lymphadenectomy. The Urologic Clinics of North America. 2010;**37**:421-434. DOI: 10.1016/j.ucl.2010.04.005

[15] Daseler EH, Anson BJ, Reinmann AF. Radical excision of the inguinal and iliac lymph glands; a study based upon 450 anatomical dissections and upon supportive clinical observations. Surgery, Gynecology & Obstetrics. 1948;**87**(6):679-694

[16] Hakenberg OW. Penile Cancer. European Association of Urology Guidelines [Internet]. 2018. Available from: https://uroweb.org/guideline/penile-cancer/ [Accessed: 2019-08-08]

[17] Flaig TM. Penile Cancer. NCCN Clinical Practice Guidelines in Oncology [Internet]. 2018. Available from: https://www.nccn.org/professionals/physician_gls/default.aspx#penile [Accessed: 2019-08-08]

Chapter 8

# Robotic Sacrocolpopexy for Treatment of Prolapse of the Apical Segment of the Vagina

*Kwang Jin Ko and Kyu-Sung Lee*


## Abstract

Abdominal sacrocolpopexy for apical prolapse repair is the gold standard treatment and is more effective and durable than the transvaginal approach. The increase in minimally invasive surgery has led to attempts at laparoscopic sacrocolpopexy, but this technique has not gained popularity due to complex procedures and a steep learning curve. Robotic sacrocolpopexy overcomes these issues and has yielded good results for more than 15 years, with equivalent outcomes and safety to open and laparoscopic sacrocolpopexy (LSC). LSC is still a useful procedure for experienced surgeons, but it is expected that robot-assisted sacrocolpopexy (RSC) will have better results overall due to the advantages of the robotic instrument. The most important advantage is that surgeons who are inexperienced with minimally invasive approaches can more readily master RSC compared to overcoming the steep learning curve of LSC.


**Keywords:** pelvic organ prolapse, robot, sacrocolpopexy

## 1. Introduction

Apical prolapse surgeries can broadly be separated into obliterative and restorative approaches. Restorative approaches can be performed transvaginally or abdominally. For patients desiring a restorative outcome, abdominal sacrocolpopexy remains the gold standard procedure, assuring superior outcomes for a variety of vaginal procedures. Sacrocolpopexy has traditionally been performed through laparotomy; however, attempts to develop minimally invasive approaches have increased to overcome the increased morbidity, longer surgery time, and longer hospital stay associated with open surgery. According to reports to date, laparoscopic sacrocolpopexy (LSC) has the advantages of a shorter hospital stay and decreased blood loss, but no benefit has been confirmed regarding surgery time, and its relatively longer learning curve has been seen as a limitation. To overcome these problems, robotic procedures began to be applied to sacrocolpopexy. After Di Marco et al. published the first study with five patients who underwent robot-assisted sacrocolpopexy (RSC) in 2004 [1], many cases have been reported, and good outcomes of RSC have been reported in apical prolapse repair. The main advantages of RSC are the three-dimensional view afforded by use of a robotic instrument, increased degrees of freedom in movement, elaborate sutures, and easy knot tying. Through the advantages of robotic surgery, LSC's technical limitations and steep learning curve can be overcome. This chapter summarizes the case results, surgical methods, and latest trends of RSC.

## 2. Efficacy

Although open sacrocolpopexy is a good treatment option for apical prolapse repair, with long-term success rates of 78–100%, it is associated with increased length of hospital stay, analgesic requirements, and cost compared with transvaginal procedures [2, 3]. To overcome these limitations, new surgical techniques, such as LSC or RSC, have been developed. Compared with open sacrocolpopexy, LSC and RSC decrease overall morbidity and have good anatomical durability [4–10]. Although LSC overcomes many of the shortcomings of open sacrocolpopexy, it is more technically challenging for those not proficient in laparoscopy. Since 2004, implementation of RLC has provided surgeons the dexterity and precision of LSC without the learning curve needed for laparoscopic skills. One of the largest prospective studies (n = 120) of RSC had an anatomical success rate of 89% over a 12-month follow-up [11]. According to a recent systematic review of LSC vs. RSC, RSC is associated with longer surgery time, increased postoperative pain, and higher cost than LSC; however, the surgical options showed similar results in terms of improvement in symptoms [12].

According to the first systematic review of RSC in 2014, the cure rate for apical prolapse was 97–100%, and the overall objective cure rate (all compartments) was 84–100% [13]. In another systematic review, the anatomic cure rate was 98.6% with a mean follow-up of 26.9 months [14]. Relapse occurred in 6.4% of the patients, with anterior, apical, and posterior recurrent prolapse rates of 3.4, 0.4, and 2.6%, respectively. The reoperation rate was 3.3%, with 0.4% caused by apical recurrent prolapse and 2.9% caused by nonapical recurrent prolapse [13]. According to a recent prospective observational study of 144 patients who received RSC and follow-up observation for at least 1 year; the cure rate of apical prolapse after 12 months was 91%; the overall cure rate was 67%; and the recurrence rates of anterior, apical, and posterior prolapse were 15.7, 0.7, and 4.3%, respectively [15]. **Table 1** reports the perioperative outcomes and cure rates.

Recently, interest has increased regarding the subjective cure rate as well as the objective anatomical cure rate, and the results of subjective evaluations are increasingly reported. Evaluation of a subjective cure, though not meeting the strict standards for anatomic success determined using POP-Q stages, emphasizes the improvement in patient's overall symptoms after the surgery and their satisfaction with the outcome. The parameters evaluated are heterogeneous but often include pelvic floor distress inventory (PFDI), pelvic floor impact questionnaire (PFIQ-7), pelvic organ prolapse/urinary incontinence sexual function questionnaire (PISQ-12), urogenital distress inventory (UDI-6), and global quality of life (QOL). Therefore, though it is necessary to note how the results are analyzed, the subjective cure rate is approximately 95% with RSC, and the satisfaction rate is high at 90–100% [13, 15, 16].

## 3. Safety and complications

According to two meta-analyses, estimated blood loss with RSC is 50–82.5 ml, and length of hospital stay is 2–2.4 days. Median surgery time is 194 min, with a wide range from 75 to 536 min, depending on the study. Hysterectomy was conducted in 33% of the patients included in the meta-analyses, and anti-incontinence

| Study | Year | Study design | Robot cases | Mean or median follow-up (month) | Objective cure rate (%) | Mean or median estimated blood loss (ml) | Mean or median hospital stay (day) | Conversion rate (%) | Mean or median (range) op time (min) | Overall complication rate (%) | Mesh extrusion (%) |
|---|---|---|---|---|---|---|---|---|---|---|---|
| Anger | 2014 | RCT | 40 | 6 | NR | 85.1 | NR | 0 | 294 (180–648) | 15 | 0 |
| Barbogilo | 2014 | RS | 127 | 12 | 92 | 127.7 | 2 | 0 | 124.2 | 10 | 2.4 |
| Belsante | 2013 | RS | 35 | 28 | 91 | 71 | 1.7 | 0 | 288 (210–390) | 14 | 3 |
| Benson | 2010 | RS | 33 | 32 | 97 | 71 | 1.1 | 0 | 227 (137–346) | 6 | 0 |
| Culligan | 2014 | PS | 143 | 12 | 84 | 51.2 | 1 | 0 | 148 (75–250) | NR | 0 |
| Elliott, D | 2006 | RS | 31 | 24 | 95 | NR | 1.03 | 3 | 186 (129–285) | 23 | 6 |
| Kramer | 2009 | RS | 21 | 25.2 | 93 | <50 | 1.1 | 0 | 194 | NR | NR |
| Louis-Sylvestre | 2013 | RS | 90 | 15.6 | 93 | NR | 3.5 | 0 | 246 (180–415) | 9 | 0 |
| Salamon | 2013 | PS | 120 | 12 | 89 | 49 | 1 | 0 | 161 | 1 | 0 |
| Seror | 2012 | PS | 20 | 15 | 98.5 | 55 | 5.1 | 5 | 125 | 30 | 0 |
| Siddiqui | 2012 | RS | 125 | 18.3 | 94 | 90 | NR | 0 | NR | 19 | 2.4 |
| Tan-Kim | 2011 | RS | 43 | 6 | 90 | 86 | 1 | 0 | 281 | NR | 5 |
| Xylinas | 2010 | RS | 12 | 19.1 | 100 | 60 | 3.4 | 0 | 144 | 0 | 0 |
| Parasio | 2011 | RCT | 40 | NR | 88 | NR | 1.8 | 9 | 257 (191–381) | 43 | 5 |

| Study | Year | Study design | Robot cases | Mean or median follow-up (month) | Objective cure rate (%) | Mean or median estimated blood loss (ml) | Mean or median hospital stay (day) | Conversion rate (%) | Mean or median (range) op time (min) | Overall complication rate (%) | Mesh extrusion (%) |
|---|---|---|---|---|---|---|---|---|---|---|---|
| Jong | 2018 | RS | 56 | 64 | 93 | 56 | 2.7 | NR | 234 | NR | 3 |
| Zanten | 2019 | PS | 188 | 12 | 91 | 25 | 1.0 | 4.3 | 145.3 | 5.3 | 2.1 |

**Table 1.**
*Summary of efficacy, perioperative outcomes, and complications in robot-assisted laparoscopic sacrocolpopexy (PS, prospective study; RCT, randomized controlled trial; RS, retrospective study).*

surgery was conducted simultaneously in 38% of patients. Therefore, it is likely that concomitant surgical procedures (including total hysterectomy, anti-incontinence procedures, and other transvaginal prolapse surgeries) contribute to the heterogeneity of surgery time [13, 14].

In the analyses above, diverse complications were reported. The overall conversion rate to open surgery was 0–8.6%, and the overall postoperative complication rate was approximately 10%. Using the Clavien-Dindo classifications for complications, 7% were Grade 1–2, <1% were Grade 3a, 2% were Grade 3b, and no Grade 4–5 complications were reported. The mesh erosion rate was 0–8% [13, 14]. Recently, a prospective, long-term study of mesh erosion after implementation of the RSC was published. Of the 69 patients analyzed, three experienced mesh erosion (3.1%) during a median 48.1 months of follow-up. Subsequent Kaplan-Meier analysis estimated an erosion rate of 5.3% in 5 years of RSC. Through additional literature analysis, the authors found that the reported erosion rate varied from 0 to 13.3% but was less than 5% in 83% of the studies, and the overall erosion rate was approximately 1.9%. Due to mesh-related complications, its use has been limited recently; however, the risk associated with transabdominally placed synthetic mesh is extremely low, and the mesh-related risk does not increase with RSC. **Table 1** lists the complications.

## 4. Surgical procedures

### 4.1 Patient positioning and port placement

The patient is placed in the lithotomy position with the Trendelenburg position to displace the bowel loops upward, providing more working space. The ports are placed in a W-shaped configuration. Generally, attached to three robot arms are one camera port and a fenestrated Grasper (Pro Grasp), robotic scissors (Hot ShearsTM), and one large needle driver; another port is used if necessary.

### 4.2 Vaginal dissection

The peritoneal cavity is assessed after robot docking. Because of the history of hysterectomy in vault prolapse patients, they may experience bowel adhesion, which must be addressed first. The mesh should be fixed to the anterior and posterior walls of the vagina; therefore, during vaginal dissection, it is important to properly detach the space between the bladder attachment to the anterior and the rectum attachment to the posterior (**Figure 1**). It is difficult to clearly distinguish the space between the cervix and bladder in patients with previous hysterectomy. Transvaginal use of a vagina manipulator aids in evaluating the anatomical structure of the surroundings. Retrograde bladder filling using a Foley catheter placed before surgery may be helpful in dissection by delineating the bladder margin. Since the plane between the anterior vaginal wall and the bladder is relatively avascular, if there is bleeding during dissection, it is typically because the wrong plane is being dissected, specifically the detrusor muscle or the vaginal muscularis.

There are no clear guidelines concerning the extent to which anterior dissection should proceed. In a systematic review of 21 randomized controlled trials, depth of vaginal dissection was a commonly described determination in the procedure that, however, involved significant heterogeneity [17]. In a survey conducted among the members of International Urogynecological Association and the American Urogynecological Society, 18% responded that they dissect only in the apex of the vagina, 56% to the mid-level of the vagina, and 25% to the level of the trigone. The

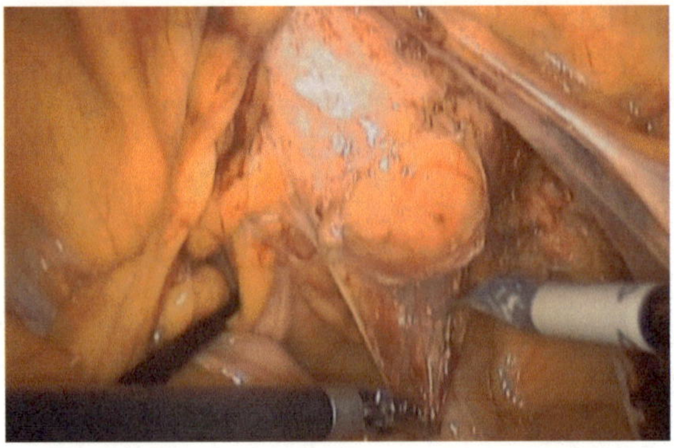

**Figure 1.**
*Vaginal wall dissection.*

generally accepted rule is to approach as close as possible to prevent recurrence but to not dissect deep to the trigone. Recently, preliminary data have been published measuring the bladder neck-mesh distance (BMD) using transvaginal ultrasound at the end of promontofixation. The BMD inversely correlated with the changes in C ($p = 0.01$) and Bp ($p = 0.04$) before and after surgery and with the complication rate ($p = 0.01$) but not with the difference in Ba. A BMD greater than 6 mm predicted the absence of postoperative *de novo* symptoms, and a short BMD predicted post-operative *de novo* symptoms such as urinary stress incontinence [18]. This indicates that BMD predicts the need for apical repair. It is necessary to conduct a well-organized study of surgical outcomes based on depth of anterior vaginal wall dissection; however, the authors judge that it is empirically sufficient to detach the anterior and posterior vaginal wall to the extent that the mesh arm is fixed (approximately the upper third of the vagina). If it is necessary to fix the mesh to the posterior vaginal wall as well, the vaginal wall should be carefully mobilized and dissected from the rectum followed by attempting to approach the recto-vagina space.

### 4.3 Presacral dissection

Presacral dissection is performed after dissection of the vaginal wall. The proximal arm of the mesh is fixed at the sacral promontory. The recommended sacral fixation point has changed due to concerns regarding hemorrhage and maintenance of the most natural vaginal axis. In the early 1970s, fixation of the mesh was typically at the level of S3/S4, but this was associated with a marked risk for hemorrhage. In 1981, Sutton et al. described fixation at the S1/S2 level for better visualization of the middle sacral artery and less risk of bleeding. Currently, the consensus is to affix the sacral arm of the mesh to the most superior point of the anterior surface of S1. However, even though attachment to the S1 region can decrease the risk of bleeding compared to other levels, it is necessary to use caution in dissection since the promontory can be anatomically unfamiliar, and there is a risk of bleeding due to the close proximity of the nerve to the surrounding blood vessels. Most of all, it is clearly necessary to be well informed regarding the anatomic relationships of the sacral promontory to other structures.

The first step in presacral dissection is retraction of the sigmoid colon to expose the peritoneum that covers the promontory. If it is difficult to expose the promontory due to surrounding bowel adhesion, adhesiolysis is performed. An important anatomical feature to aid in finding the promontory is the pulsating right common iliac artery (**Figure 2**). Starting from this point, the peritoneum in the most prominent region of the endoscopic view is opened first. It may be difficult for inexperienced practitioners to find the exact position when the peritoneum is covered. In patients with thick presacral fat pads, it is especially difficult to identify the surrounding structures. In these cases, the right ureter may be a useful landmark as it is found approximately 30 mm lateral to the sacral promontory. Therefore, measuring 30 mm medial to the right ureter along the pelvic brim should allow the surgeon to identify the most likely location of the sacral promontory [19]. The peritoneum is then dissected, and the incision is typically extended to the cul-de-sac region to make space to cover the mesh. However, we prefer to make space by tunneling into the region of vaginal dissection instead of using a long incision in the posterior peritoneum. This is because tunneling can lessen the inconvenience of subsequent closure of the peritoneum.

### 4.4 Mesh and fixation

In an effort to decrease the morbidity associated with open sacrocolpopexy, RSC has rapidly gained popularity because it decreases the difficulty with laparoscopic knot tying and aids in sacral dissection due to three-dimensional visualization. However, variables in surgical technique include amount of vaginal dissection, type of mesh, number or location of sutures that should be placed to secure the suspending mesh, retroperitonealization of the mesh, and cervix preservation.

The chemical makeup of the synthetic material used in the mesh does not affect the success of the procedure. However, pore size is important in the ability of the host to eliminate bacteria. Macrophages and leukocytes can enter macroporous mesh and prevent infection. Fiber composition is interconnected with pore size; in multifilament mesh material, there are microporous interstices between the filaments. Thus, Type 1 mesh (i.e., macroporous and monofilament) should be used. We use pre-fashioned Y-shaped DynaMesh®-PRS, which is a polyvinylidene fluoride (PVDF) monofilament material. The use of pre-fashioned Y-shaped mesh compared to a self-fashioned mesh does not have a major impact on the success rate of the surgery [20]. The mesh is fixed to the anterior and posterior vaginal wall with multiple sutures to distribute tension on the vagina (**Figure 3**). The choice of suture material, suture gauge, and number of sutures may vary highly depending on surgical approach [17]. The traditional open sacrocolpopexy uses a nonabsorbable suture to prevent detaching the mesh from the vagina and sacral promontory and decreasing the risk of mesh exposure and suture erosion. In a study of RSC with a median follow-up of 33 months, the use of absorbable sutures for both vaginal and sacral mesh attachment was effective, and the 3-year rate of survival without repeat prolapse surgery was 93%. However, there was no benefit of the risk of

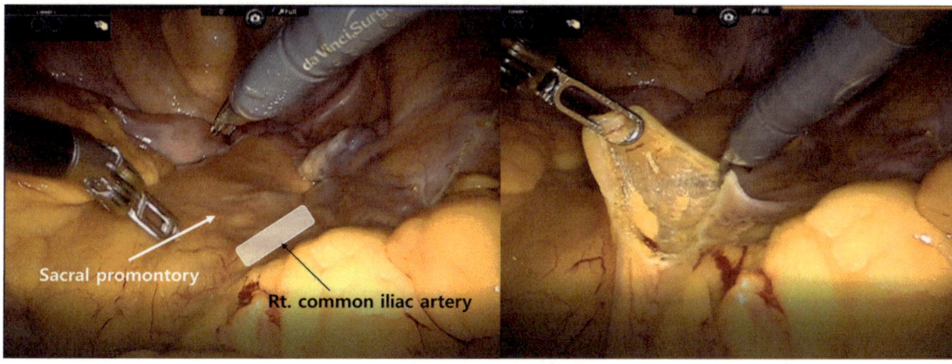


**Figure 2.**
*Anatomy of sacral promontory (left) and presacral dissection (right).*

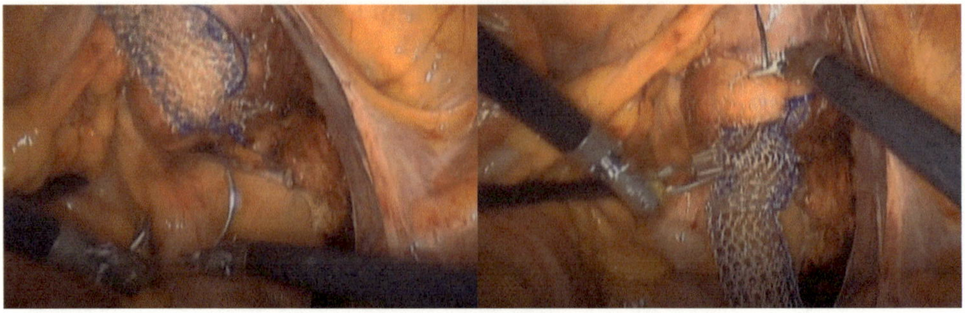

**Figure 3.**
*Fix the mesh to the anterior and posterior vaginal wall.*

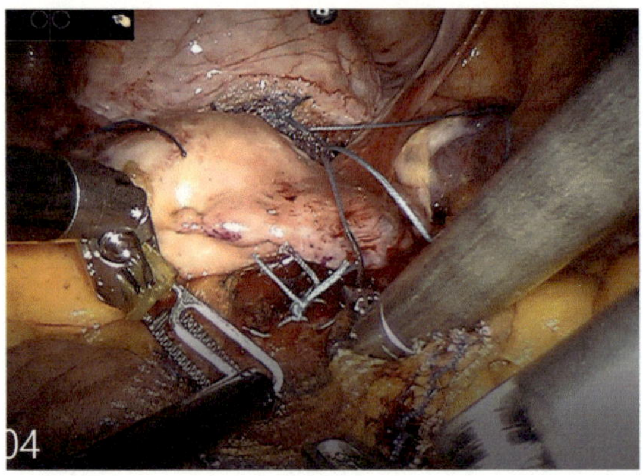

**Figure 4.**
*Fixation of the proximal arm of mesh.*

mesh erosion [21]. Although the evidence is still lacking, it is unlikely that absorbable sutures are a risk factor for mesh detachment. Further studies are needed to determine the proper location, number, and type of suture. Recently, a barbed absorbable suture material has been used in a continuous running suture along the vaginal wall with good results. Tan-Kim et al. [22]conducted a randomized study comparing non-barbed, interrupted sutures to barbed sutures (Quill™) for anchoring mesh to the vaginal wall during RSC. Among the patients, the non-barbed suture group had significantly longer surgery times than the barbed suture group (42 vs. 29 minutes, $p < 0.001$), and there was no significant difference in anatomic failure between the two groups at 12 months postoperation. Another retrospective study reported the outcomes of 20 patients who underwent RSC using barbed, delayed-absorption sutures (3–0 V-Loc 180, Covidien) to fix the mesh to the vaginal wall. There was no recurrence of apical prolapse or mesh exposure during the 1-year follow-up [23].

The proximal arm of the mesh should be fixed in the sacral promontory (**Figure 4**). At this time, the tension of the mesh should be adjusted while the prolapse is restored using the vaginal manipulator. Excessive tension may cause pain or irritative bladder symptoms after surgery. The mesh is sutured to the anterior longitudinal ligament overlying the sacrum with 2–5 sutures. As the endoscopic approach becomes more common, reports of postoperative discitis are gradually increasing. This is primarily caused by penetration of the L5-S1 disc; therefore, surgeons should ensure attachment to the S1 body below the disc. According to a study of spinal magnetic resonance images of subjects in the supine position, the most prominent point of the promontory was the L5-S1 disc in 73% of cases, and the S1 body was located within 5 mm inferior to the promontory in 100% of the images reviewed [24]. Unless the position of the S1 body can be confirmed, surgeons should take into account the thickness of the anterior longitudinal ligament, which ranges from 1 to 2 mm, and should avoid deep suture bites that may penetrate into the disc.

It is optimal to suture the peritoneum after mesh fixation. A few reports have stated that they found no complications even though peritoneal closure was not conducted; however, it is preferable to perform this step to prevent bowel adhesion or intraabdominal mesh complications.

### 4.5 Single-port approach

The "single-port approach" is a sign of a new era in the field of minimally invasive surgeries with good cosmetic results and reduced patient morbidity compared with multiport surgery. Though single-port robotic surgery is in the early stage of application, it has been implemented in various surgical fields. Since 2017, a few reports on single-port RSC have been published and are being accepted as feasible techniques [25–28]. In 2017, Matanes et al. [27] reported the first 25 cases of single-port RSC. They demonstrated significant decreases in median total operative and console times (226 minutes for the first 15 cases vs. 156 minutes for the next 10 cases), which was in the same range as that reported for the initial experience with multiport access. There were no intraoperative adverse events. One case of small bowel obstruction required reoperation; however, that patient did not receive retroperitonealized mesh. That event altered the surgeon's approach with all subsequent patients, who had mesh covered by the peritoneum. Recently, Liu et al. [26] published another case series of single-port RSC with a modified technique. They used retroperitoneal tunneling techniques and asserted that they could more easily perform a single-port approach as a result. A retroperitoneal tunnel was created by undermining the peritoneum with an articulated needle driver. The needle driver was placed in the peritoneal opening over the sacral promontory, and the tunnel was created just medial to the right uterosacral ligament in the direction of the vaginal vault. The tunnel was created using forward pressure and a sweeping motion to create a space within the retroperitoneum. This allowed easier adjustment and maintenance of mesh tension during placement of sutures in the sacral promontory compared with opening the entire retroperitoneal space and may reduce operative time and adhesion formation.

## 5. Conclusions

Despite the limitation that various methods are used by individual surgeons for evaluating the outcomes of pelvic organ prolapse repair and other surgical procedures, the use of RSC in apical prolapse repair has led to good long-term results in terms of efficacy and safety over the last 15 years. LSC is still a useful procedure for experienced surgeons, but it is expected that RSC will have better results overall due to the advantages of the robotic instrument. The most important advantage is that surgeons who are inexperienced with minimally invasive approaches can more readily master RSC compared to overcoming the steep learning curve of LSC.

## Author details

Kwang Jin Ko[1] and Kyu-Sung Lee[2,3]*

1 Department of Urology, Kangnam Sacred Heart Hospital, Hallym University College of Medicine, Seoul, Republic of Korea

2 Department of Urology, Samsung Medical Center, Sungkyunkwan University School of Medicine, Seoul, Republic of Korea

3 Biomedical Engineering Research Center, Samsung Medical Center, Seoul, Republic of Korea

*Address all correspondence to: ksleedr@skku.edu

## References

[1] Di Marco DS, Chow GK, Gettman MT, Elliott DS. Robotic-assisted laparoscopic sacrocolpopexy for treatment of vaginal vault prolapse. Urology. 2004;**63**(2):373-376

[2] Lee RK, Mottrie A, Payne CK, Waltregny D. A review of the current status of laparoscopic and robot-assisted sacrocolpopexy for pelvic organ prolapse. European Urology. 2014;**65**(6):1128-1137

[3] Nygaard IE, McCreery R, Brubaker L, Connolly A, Cundiff G, Weber AM, et al. Abdominal sacrocolpopexy: A comprehensive review. Obstetrics and Gynecology. 2004;**104**(4):805-823

[4] Anger JT, Mueller ER, Tarnay C, Smith B, Stroupe K, Rosenman A, et al. Robotic compared with laparoscopic sacrocolpopexy: A randomized controlled trial. Obstetrics and Gynecology. 2014;**123**(1):5-12

[5] Costantini E, Mearini L, Lazzeri M, Bini V, Nunzi E, di Biase M, et al. Laparoscopic versus abdominal Sacrocolpopexy: A randomized, controlled trial. The Journal of Urology. 2016;**196**(1):159-165

[6] Freeman RM, Pantazis K, Thomson A, Frappell J, Bombieri L, Moran P, et al. A randomised controlled trial of abdominal versus laparoscopic sacrocolpopexy for the treatment of post-hysterectomy vaginal vault prolapse: LAS study. International Urogynecology Journal. 2013;**24**(3):377-384

[7] Geller EJ, Siddiqui NY, Wu JM, Visco AG. Short-term outcomes of robotic sacrocolpopexy compared with abdominal sacrocolpopexy. Obstetrics and Gynecology. 2008;**112**(6):1201-1206

[8] Nosti PA, Umoh Andy U, Kane S, White DE, Harvie HS, Lowenstein L, et al. Outcomes of abdominal and minimally invasive sacrocolpopexy: A retrospective cohort study. Female Pelvic Medicine & Reconstructive Surgery. 2014;**20**(1):33-37

[9] Paraiso MF, Jelovsek JE, Frick A, Chen CC, Barber MD. Laparoscopic compared with robotic sacrocolpopexy for vaginal prolapse: A randomized controlled trial. Obstetrics and Gynecology. 2011;**118**(5):1005-1013

[10] Siddiqui NY, Geller EJ, Visco AG. Symptomatic and anatomic 1-year outcomes after robotic and abdominal sacrocolpopexy. American Journal of Obstetrics and Gynecology. 2012;**206**(5):435.e1-435.e5

[11] Salamon CG, Lewis C, Priestley J, Gurshumov E, Culligan PJ. Prospective study of an ultra-lightweight polypropylene Y mesh for robotic sacrocolpopexy. International Urogynecology Journal. 2013;**24**(8):1371-1375

[12] Pan K, Zhang Y, Wang Y, Wang Y, Xu H. A systematic review and meta-analysis of conventional laparoscopic sacrocolpopexy versus robot-assisted laparoscopic sacrocolpopexy. International Journal of Gynaecology and Obstetrics: The Official Organ of the International Federation of Gynaecology and Obstetrics. 2016;**132**(3):284-291

[13] Serati M, Bogani G, Sorice P, Braga A, Torella M, Salvatore S, et al. Robot-assisted sacrocolpopexy for pelvic organ prolapse: A systematic review and meta-analysis of comparative studies. European Urology. 2014;**66**(2):303-318

[14] Hudson CO, Northington GM, Lyles RH, Karp DR. Outcomes of robotic sacrocolpopexy: A systematic review and meta-analysis. Female Pelvic Medicine & Reconstructive Surgery. 2014;**20**(5):252-260

[15] van Zanten F, Schraffordt Koops SE, O'Sullivan OE, Lenters E, Broeders I, O'Reilly BA. Robot-assisted surgery for the management of apical prolapse: A bi-Centre prospective cohort study. BJOG: An International Journal of Obstetrics and Gynaecology. 2019;**126**(8):1065-1073

[16] Jong K, Klein T, Zimmern PE. Long-term outcomes of robotic mesh sacrocolpopexy. Journal of Robotic Surgery. 2018;**12**(3):455-460

[17] Moroni RM, Juliato CRT, Cosson M, Giraudet G, Brito LGO. Does sacrocolpopexy present heterogeneity in its surgical technique? A systematic review. Neurourology and Urodynamics. 2018;**37**(8):2335-2345

[18] Habib N, Centini G, Pizzoferrato AC, Bui C, Argay I, Bader G. Laparoscopic promontofixation: Where to stop the anterior dissection? Medical Hypotheses. 2019;**124**:60-63

[19] McCullough M, Valceus J, Downes K, Hoyte L. The ureter as a landmark for robotic sacrocolpopexy. Female Pelvic Medicine & Reconstructive Surgery. 2012;**18**(3):162-164

[20] Ferrando CA, Paraiso MFR. A prospective randomized trial comparing Restorelle Y mesh and flat mesh for laparoscopic and robotic-assisted laparoscopic Sacrocolpopexy. Female Pelvic Medicine & Reconstructive Surgery. 2019;**25**(2):83-87

[21] Linder BJ, Anand M, Klingele CJ, Trabuco EC, Gebhart JB, Occhino JA. Outcomes of robotic Sacrocolpopexy using only absorbable suture for mesh fixation. Female Pelvic Medicine & Reconstructive Surgery. 2017;**23**(1):13-16

[22] Tan-Kim J, Nager CW, Grimes CL, Luber KM, Lukacz ES, Brown HW, et al. A randomized trial of vaginal mesh attachment techniques for minimally invasive sacrocolpopexy. International Urogynecology Journal. 2015;**26**(5):649-656

[23] Borahay MA, Oge T, Walsh TM, PatelPR, RodriguezAM, KilicGS. Outcomes of robotic sacrocolpopexy using barbed delayed absorbable sutures. Journal of Minimally Invasive Gynecology. 2014;**21**(3):412-416

[24] Abernethy M, Vasquez E, Kenton K, Brubaker L, Mueller E. Where do we place the sacrocolpopexy stitch? A magnetic resonance imaging investigation. Female Pelvic Medicine & Reconstructive Surgery. 2013;**19**(1):31-33

[25] Guan X, Ma Y, Gisseman J, Kleithermes C, Liu J. Robotic single-site Sacrocolpopexy using barbed suture anchoring and peritoneal tunneling technique: Tips and tricks. Journal of Minimally Invasive Gynecology. 2017;**24**(1):12-13

[26] Liu J, Bardawil E, Zurawin RK, Wu J, Fu H, Orejuela F, et al. Robotic single-site Sacrocolpopexy with retroperitoneal tunneling. JSLS: Journal of the Society of Laparoendoscopic Surgeons. 2018;**22**(3):e2018.00009

[27] Matanes E, Lauterbach R, Mustafa-Mikhail S, Amit A, Wiener Z, Lowenstein L. Single port robotic assisted Sacrocolpopexy: Our experience with the first 25 cases. Female Pelvic Medicine & Reconstructive Surgery. 2017;**23**(3):e14-ee8

[28] Lowenstein L, Matanes E, Burke YZ. Surgical technique for robot-assisted Sacrocolpopexy performed via a single port. Urology. 2017;**103**:272

Chapter 9

# Robot-Assisted Kidney Transplantation

*Karel Decaestecker, Angelo Territo, Riccardo Campi, Benjamin Van Parys, Giulio Bevilacqua, Liesbeth Desender and Alberto Breda*

## Abstract

Robot-assisted kidney transplantation (RAKT) has recently been introduced to reduce the morbidity of open kidney transplantation (KT). Robot-assisted surgery has been able to overcome many of the limitations of classical laparoscopy, certainly in complex and technically demanding procedures, such as vascular and ureteral anastomosis. Since the first RAKT in 2010, this technique has been standardized and evaluated in highly experienced robot and KT centers around the world. In Europe, the European Association of Urology Robotic Urology Section (ERUS) created an RAKT working group in 2016 in order to prospectively follow the outcomes of RAKT. When performed by surgeons with both robotic and KT experience, RAKT has been proven to be safe and reproducible in selected cases and yield excellent graft function with a low complication rate. Multiple institutions have now adopted RAKT, and its use will likely increase in the near future. However, structured training and proctoring will be mandatory for those embarking on RAKT in order to help them negotiate the learning curve and avoid technical mistakes. This chapter will describe RAKT from living and deceased donors and its application in kidney autotransplantation (KAT).

**Keywords:** kidney transplantation, living donor, deceased donor, autotransplantation, robot-assisted kidney transplantation, robot-assisted kidney autotransplantation, robot-assisted, robotic

## 1. Introduction

Kidney transplantation (KT) is considered the preferred treatment for patients with end-stage renal disease (ESRD) owing to the greater survival rate and better quality of life in comparison to hemodialysis [1]. To date, the open approach has been the gold standard in KT, despite its invasiveness and high morbidity. Minimally invasive surgery may be a good alternative to reduce the morbidity associated with the open approach, especially in immunocompromised and fragile KT patients and even more in obese recipients who are known to have a higher complication rate.

Minimally invasive surgery (using a pure laparoscopic or a robot-assisted approach) offers significant benefits to patients compared to open surgery, including improved peri- and postoperative outcomes, such as shorter hospital stay, less postoperative pain, shorter convalescence period, fewer wound infections, and better cosmetic results [2]. Robot-assisted surgery has been able to overcome many of the limitations of classical laparoscopy, especially in complex and technically demanding surgical procedures, such as reconstruction or vascular and ureteral anastomosis. This has been attributed to the superb three-dimensional vision, magnification (12×), control of the camera by the surgeon, elimination of hand tremor, and seven degrees of freedom of movement [3].

This chapter will describe the history, technique and results of robot-assisted kidney transplantation (RAKT) from living donors and deceased donors, and also its application in kidney autotransplantation (KAT).

## 2. Robot-assisted kidney transplantation (RAKT): living donor

### 2.1 History and background

#### *2.1.1 Living donor nephrectomy*

Open donor nephrectomies were carried out for nearly 50 years until the introduction of laparoscopy in 1995 by Ratner et al. [4]. Since its first description in 1995, the laparoscopic approach for donor nephrectomy has demonstrated to improve peri- and postoperative outcomes such as blood loss, pain, hospital stay, as well as cosmetic results, when compared to open surgery. In 2001, the first series of robot-assisted laparoscopic donor nephrectomy, using the da Vinci® Surgical System (Intuitive Surgical, Sunnyvale, CA, USA), was reported by the Group of the University of Illinois (Chicago) [5]. They demonstrated that robot-assisted nephrectomy is feasible, safe, and reproducible, providing similar results in comparison to the laparoscopic approach [6, 7]. Nowadays, around 40% of all KT in the USA and around 20% of all KT in Europe are performed with living donors. Every year, the ratio of "emotionally related" living donors to genetically related living donors increases slightly, with most of the living donors currently being family members [8]. In comparison with KT from deceased donors, KT from living donors provides several advantages in terms of long-term patient survival, earlier graft function, longer graft survival, less aggressive immunosuppressive regimens, and reduced waiting lists [9]. When a living donor has two equally functioning kidneys, the left kidney is preferred for donation as the left renal vein is longer compared to the right renal vein. When the kidney function of both kidneys is different, the lesser functioning kidney is used for donation, in order to limit the risks for the donor. Many concerns have been raised regarding the use of the right kidney for living donation, but literature suggests that right laparoscopic donor nephrectomy is feasible and results in good graft function [10, 11].

#### *2.1.2 Living donor kidney transplantation*

RAKT has recently been introduced to reduce the morbidity of open KT. Since the first RAKT in 2010 by Giulianotti et al. [12] in the USA, this technique has been standardized and evaluated in highly experienced robot and KT centers around the world. In 2014 Menon et al. [13] standardized the technique with the transperitoneal approach and regional hypothermia known as the Vattikuti-Medanta technique. The authors highlighted that RAKT is a safe technique with possible advantages such as low intra- and postoperative complications, better cosmetic results, and superlative vision that could result in better quality of the vascular and ureteral anastomoses. The first two European pure RAKTs were performed in July 2015 by Breda et al. [14] and Doumerc et al. [15]. In 2016, the European Association of Urology (EAU) formed the EAU Robotic Urology Section (ERUS) RAKT working group in order to prospectively follow the outcomes of RAKT. Breda et al. [16] published the largest multicenter series of RAKT to date (120 patients). Angelo Territo et al. [17] addressed the functional results of RAKT from living donors at 1-year follow-up, and Vignolini et al. [18] developed a RAKT program with grafts from deceased donors. Siena et al. [19] described the technique for RAKT in grafts with multiple vessels. The feasibility of RAKT in children was described by the Ghent University group by Spinoit et al. [20].

## 2.2 Operative technique

### *2.2.1 Living donor nephrectomy*

To date, several techniques are described for living donor nephrectomy, including open surgery, pure laparoscopy, hand-assisted laparoscopy, and robot-assisted surgery [21–23]. The most commonly used technique is the minimally invasive transperitoneal laparoscopic approach. According to the literature, laparoscopic surgery for living donor nephrectomy achieves similar functional results compared to open and robot-assisted living donor nephrectomy, being equally safe for the donor. Robot-assisted surgery offers clear advantages over conventional laparoscopy, thanks to the use of EndoWrist instruments, three-dimensional view, enhanced visualization of the operative field (12x), and, possibly, a shorter learning curve [21, 24]. Open nephrectomy for donation may offer an advantage in challenging cases such as grafts with multiple vessels and/or vascular anomalies and prior abdominal surgery. Furthermore, the open approach may be preferred in centers with low experience in laparoscopy and/or a low case volume of living donor nephrectomies [25] (**Figure 1**).

### *2.2.2 Back table preparation*

After robot-assisted/laparoscopic living donor nephrectomy, the preparation of the kidney is performed at the back table close to the operating bed. First, the graft is placed in a basin with slushed ice and perfused with 1 liter of storage solution (Celsior®, or Custodiol®, or Institut Georges Lopez-1®). Next, the graft vessels

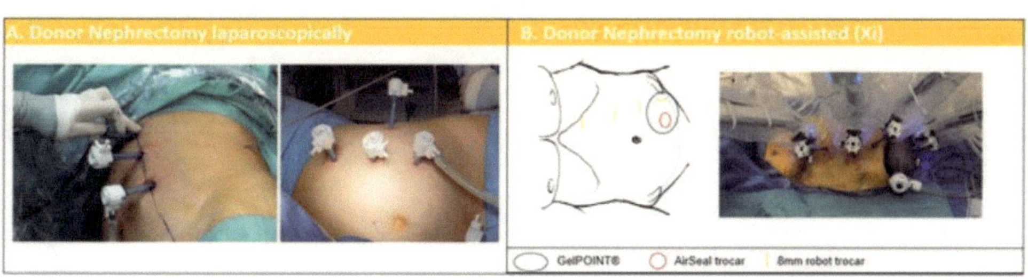


**Figure 1.**
*Trocar placement and patient positioning for nephrectomy during RAKT on living donors. (A) Laparoscopically: patient positioned in lateral decubitus, linear port configuration along the pararectal line, with the camera placed at the most cephalic position (at the 12th rib level). (B) Robot-assisted: patient positioned in lateral decubitus; GelPOINT® device at the level of the ipsilateral fossa through a 6 cm Pfannenstiel incision; a 15-mm AirSeal trocar is placed in the device to introduce endovascular stapler and the 15-mm EndoCatch bag for organ extraction. An additional trocar is used to raise the kidney during the section of the vessels.*

are carefully dissected. If the donor kidney has multiple arteries or veins, a vascular reconstruction can be performed. Siena et al. [19] demonstrated that RAKT is possible using grafts with multiple vessels. The ureter can be pre-stented with a double-J if preferred. Subsequently, the kidney is wrapped in a gauze filled with slushed ice, with the artery and vein brought out through an opening in the gauze (**Figure 2**). The aim is to keep the donor kidney at a constant low temperature after insertion in the abdominal cavity, until the vascular anastomoses are finished, and the kidney is reperfused. In addition, the gauze can prevent potential graft injury from manipulation with the robot arms. To keep the graft temperature below 20°C intracorporeally, ice is added through the GelPOINT® (Applied Medical, Rancho Santa Margarita, CA, USA) every 15 min.

### *2.2.3 Robot-assisted living donor kidney transplantation*

#### *2.2.3.1 Patient and trocar positioning*

When using the da Vinci Si® or X® system, the patient is positioned in lithotomy position according to the Vattikuti-Medanta technique [26]. When the da Vinci Xi® system is used, the patient is positioned in dorsal decubitus. A 20–30° Trendelenburg position is recommended. The required robotic instruments are monopolar scissors, Potts scissors, bipolar forceps, prograsp forceps, large needle driver, black diamond micro-forceps, and bulldog clamps. A 12 mm camera port is inserted in the supra-umbilical area, and a pneumoperitoneum is created. Veress needle puncture, optical trocar access, or the Hasson technique can also be used for access to the abdomen and creation of a pneumoperitoneum. The open approach (Hasson technique) has been reported to result in fewer complications [27]. Three extra robotic 8 mm ports are placed under vision, and the robot is docked.

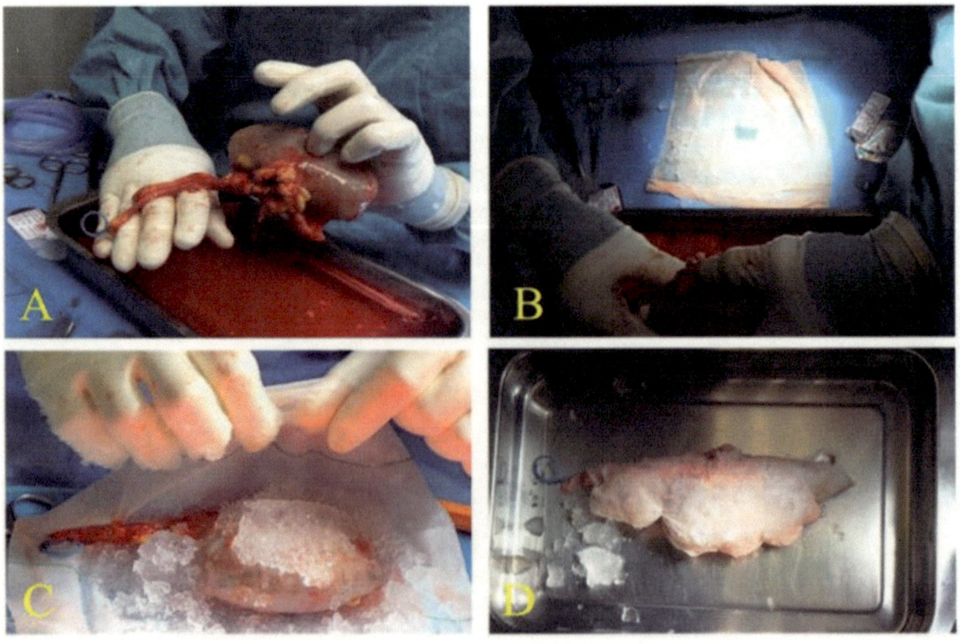


**Figure 2.**
*Preparation of the kidney graft after nephrectomy during RAKT from living donors. (A) Ureteral double J stent is placed in the graft. (B) A central hole in the gauze from which the artery and vein are outside. (C and D) The graft is wrapped in a gauze jacket filled with ice slush.*

Minimal changes in port placement are related according to the robotic system used (**Figure 3**). A GelPOINT® device replaces the camera trocar through a 6–8 cm (four fingers) periumbilical incision (**Figure 4**) once the transplant bed preparation has been performed. Alternatively, the GelPOINT® device can be introduced from the beginning through a 6–8 cm periumbilical incision, containing the camera and an assistant port. This GelPOINT® device is used to introduce the graft in the abdominal cavity (**Figure 4**) and allows for insertion of slushed ice (± 200 ml) via modified Toomey syringes into the abdominal cavity, surrounding the graft surface with the intent to achieve regional hypothermia (i.e., low constant temperature (<20°C) of the graft). Additionally, GelPOINT® is a useful device for fast hand introduction if needed (i.e., in case of massive bleeding). In selected cases, the graft can be introduced transvaginal as described by few authors [15]. The AirSeal® (Conmed, Utica, NY, USA) system might be used in order to maintain a stable and low-pressure pneumoperitoneum at 8 mmHg.

*2.2.3.2 Transplant bed preparation*

Accurate dissection of the external iliac vessels is performed. Subsequently, the bladder is prepared for ureteral reimplantation. A retroperitoneal pouch is created by incision of the peritoneum following a transverse line above the level of the appendix and mobilization of the peritoneal flaps. These will be used to cover (retroperitonealize) the graft once the vascular anastomosis is completed. Although RAKT is a transperitoneal approach, retroperitonealization of the kidney is performed to avoid pedicle torsion and to enable future graft biopsies.

*2.2.3.3 Venous and arterial anastomosis*

After clamping of the external iliac vein with robotic bulldog clamps and the distal clamp followed by the proximal clamp, a longitudinal venotomy using cold scissors is performed. An end-to-side anastomosis between the graft renal vein and the external iliac vein is created, using a 6/0 Gore-Tex® CV-6 TTc-9 or THc-12 needle (W.L. Gore and Associates Inc., Flagstaff, AZ, USA) continuous suture. At the proximal angle, the suture is tied to secure the posterior wall of the anastomosis watertight and to avoid stenosis, and then the continuous suture is completed until the distal angle. Prior to finishing the anastomosis, the lumen is flushed with heparinized solution using a 4.8 Fr ureteric catheter. The catheter may be pulled out by the assistant from outside the abdomen while the surgeon

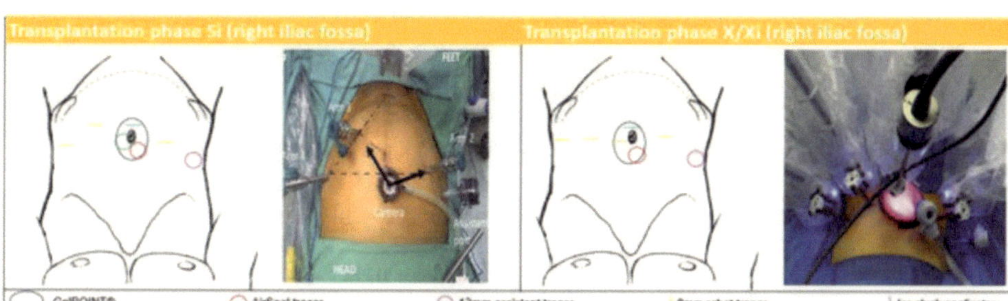


**Figure 3.**
*Trocar placement and patient positioning for RAKT for Si/X/Xi in the right iliac fossa. Patient repositioned in dorsal decubitus, legs in Allen stirrups, table in 20–30° Trendelenburg; GelPOINT® device at the level of the umbilicus through a 6–8 cm vertical peri-umbilical incision; camera trocar and ice applicator in the GelPOINT® (eventually with 12 mm AirSeal® port); 3–8 mm robotic trocars in the lower abdomen, 2 in the left fossa and 1 in the right iliac fossa.*

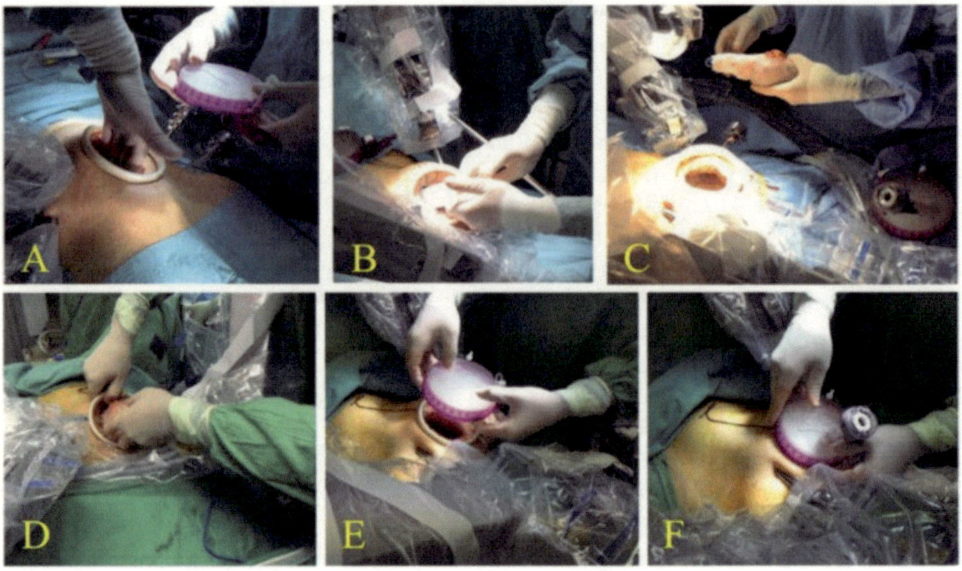


**Figure 4.**
*Introduction of the kidney and ice through the Gel-POINT®. (A) The GelPOINT® device is placed through a 6 cm (four fingers) incision. (B) Ice slush is introduced in the abdominal cavity using modified Toomey syringes. (C and D) The graft is introduced into the abdominal cavity. (E and F) Once the graft is inside, Gel-POINT® cup is inserted to close the abdomen.*

tightens the knot to secure the anastomosis (**Figure 5**). Next, the graft vein is clamped, and the bulldog clamps are removed from the external iliac vein and positioned on the external iliac artery, first proximally and then distally. The artery may be incised with the cold scissors or a scalpel at the 1–2 o'clock position. Arteriotomy may be completed using a laparoscopic aortic punch to transform the linear arteriotomy into a circular one. In both arterial and venous anastomosis, the anastomosis is started by passing the needle in the external iliac vessel in an outside-inside direction and then inside-outside through the graft vessel (**Figure 6**). For the venous anastomosis, the knot is tied now, and the needle is then passed outside-inside through the renal vein to start the running suture. For the arterial anastomosis, the suture is not tied yet (as for the venous anastomosis), and the needle is passed through the graft artery outside-inside before tying the suture to a loop that is left outside. This is done to prevent a difficult first needle passing in a small arterial lumen. After completing the arterial anastomosis, a clamp is positioned on the graft artery while the external iliac artery is declamped. If no sign of leakage (bleeding) is observed, the graft vein and artery are declamped. The evaluation of the graft perfusion is primarily visual: pink colorization, a pulsatile graft artery, filling of the renal vein, and small bleedings from the renal capsule and urine output are signs of perfusion. Doppler ultrasound evaluation (drop-in ultrasound probe linked to TilePro™ function of the da Vinci Surgical System) is recommended to verify adequate perfusion of the graft.

*2.2.3.4 Ureteroneocystostomy*

After flipping the kidney on the psoas and retroperitonealization of the graft, the ureteroneocystostomy is performed according to the Lich-Gregoire technique using a Monocryl or PDS 5/0 (Ethicon Inc., Cincinnati, OH, USA) continuous

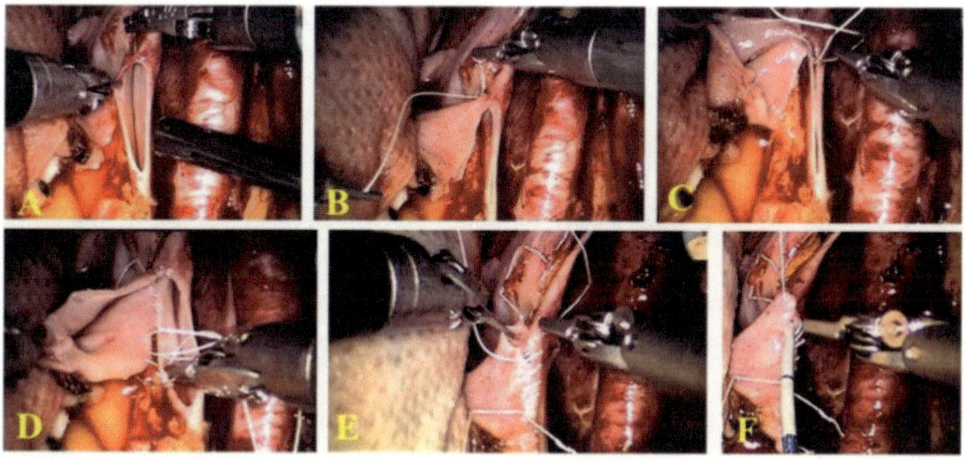


**Figure 5.**
*Overview of the main steps for venous anastomosis during RAKT from living donors. (A) The graft renal vein is anastomosed in an end-to-side continuous fashion to the external iliac vein using a 6/0 Gore-Tex®. (B and C) At cranial angle, the suture is knotted to fix the posterior wall of the anastomosis. (D and E) The running suture is completed at the caudal angle. (F) Before completing the anastomosis, the lumen is flushed with heparinized solution using a 4.8 Fr ureteral catheter.*

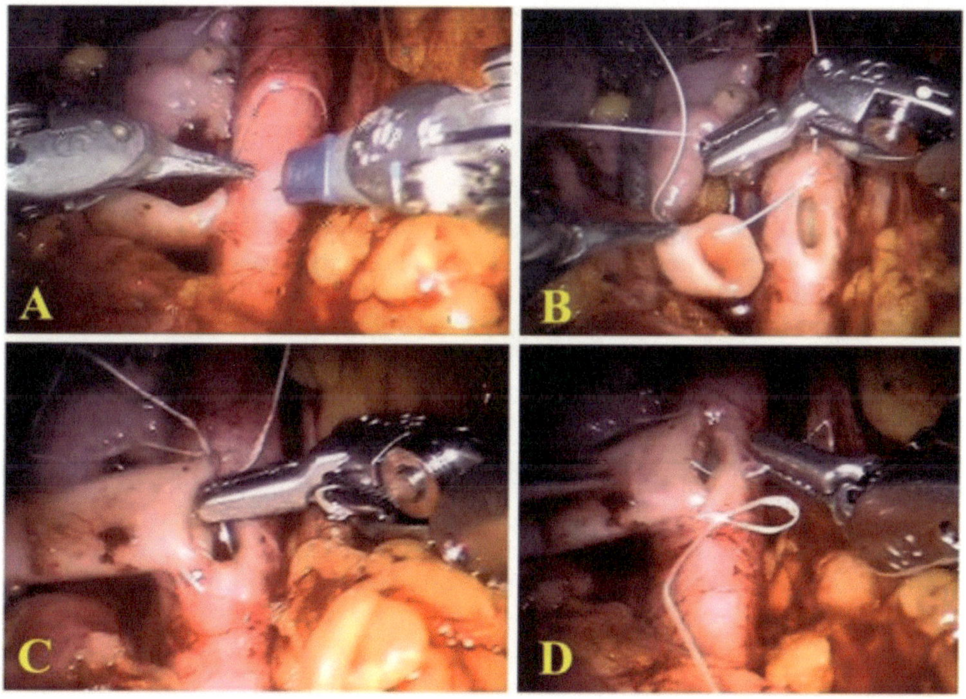


**Figure 6.**
*Overview of the main steps for arterial anastomosis during RAKT from living donors. (A) The robotic scalpel is used to make a linear incision on the iliac artery, converting it in circular hole with a laparoscopic vascular punch. (B) The running suture is carried out using a 6/0 Gore-Tex®; particularly in the caudal tying of an arterial anastomosis, the needle is passed in the external iliac vessel in an outside-inside direction, then outside-inside through the graft vessel. (C and D) The running suture is completed at the caudal angle.*

suture (**Figure 7**). Care is taken to construct an adequate detrusor tunnel as anti-reflux mechanism. A double-J stent is inserted to protect the anastomosis. The stent can be removed after 3 weeks.

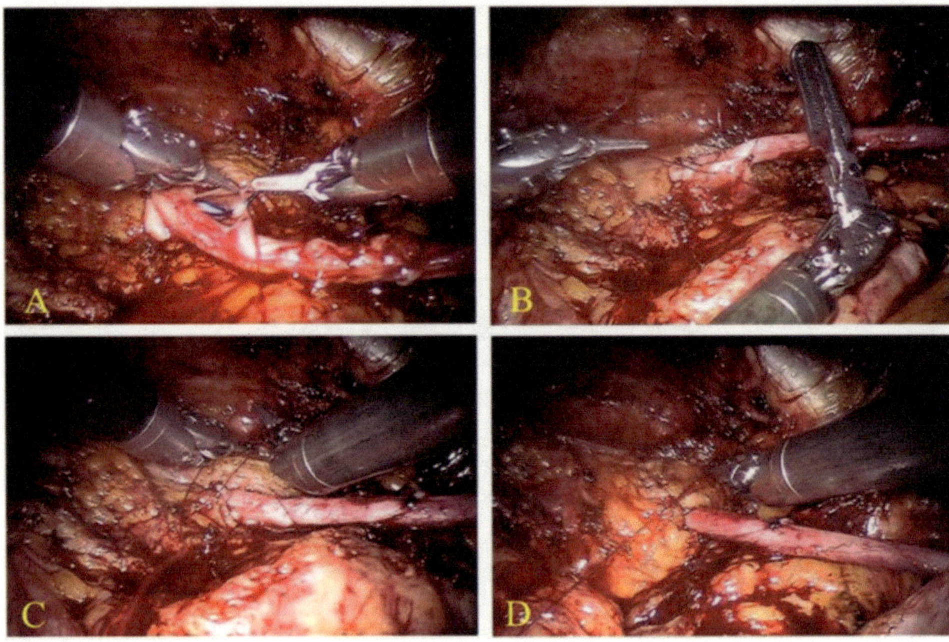

**Figure 7.**
*Ureteroneocystostomy performed according to the Lich-Gregoir technique. In (A) and (B) running suture between ureteral and bladder mucosa using 5-0 Monocryl. In (C) and (D) the details of the anti-reflux tunnel.*

### 2.3 Results

After reporting a single center experience on 17 cases of RAKT from living donation [28], the European Experience in RAKT was published in 2018. One hundred twenty cases were prospectively collected in eight centers across Europe [16]. The authors demonstrated the low complication rate (at 1 month follow-up) while maintaining excellent graft function (median eGFR at 30 days was 58 ml/min) and cosmetic results (**Figure 8**). Three cases of graft loss due to arterial thrombosis during the first postoperative week were reported in these series (2.5%). This complication might be associated with technical errors during the learning curve. Territo et al. [17] demonstrated that the functional results at 1-year follow-up were not statistically different from the functional results at 1-month follow-up. The complication rate remained low. To date, there are no studies available comparing RAKT with the conventional open approach. However, an increasing body of evidence confirms that RAKT is at least non-inferior to open KT regarding both patient and graft survival [16, 29].

## 3. Robot-assisted kidney transplantation (RAKT): deceased donor

### 3.1 Background

The vast majority of RAKT worldwide has been performed from living donors, raising concerns regarding the generalizability of RAKT outcomes in the broader and more challenging scenario of deceased donors.

While it has been shown that the learning curve for elective RAKT (i.e., living donor RAKT) may be minimal for surgeons with extensive experience in robotic surgery (regardless of their background in open KT) [30, 31], RAKT

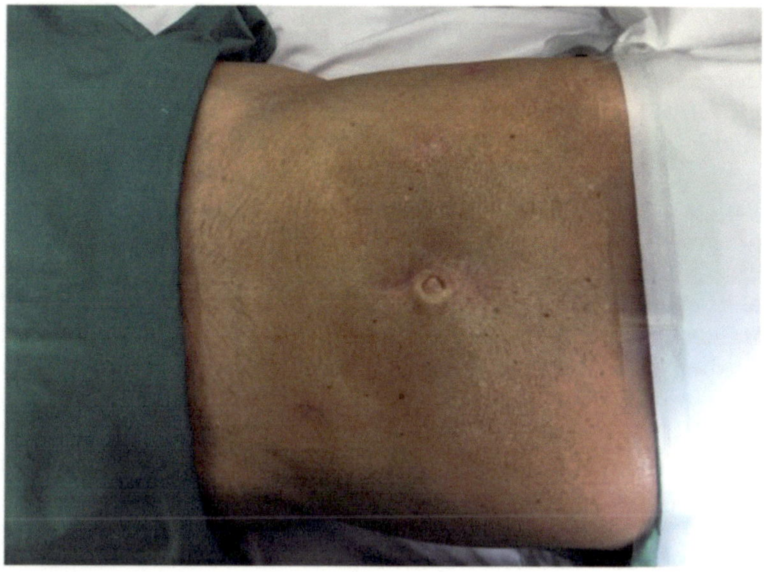

**Figure 8.**
*Esthetic results of RAKT 3 months later.*

from deceased donors has unique technical and logistical challenges. Indeed, due to the timeframe of organ preservation, it can be considered an unforeseeable "emergency" robotic procedure, which requires a structured multidisciplinary framework.

### 3.2 Development of a structured RAKT program from deceased donors

To fill this gap and move the field forward, the University of Florence group has recently developed a RAKT program from deceased donors aiming to safely and progressively increase the pool of patients who may benefit from minimally invasive KT [18].

The cornerstones of this program are as follows: (a) an extensive experience in open KT (n > 1100 KTs from 1991) and robotic urologic surgery (>4000 procedures from 2010, including radical prostatectomy, radical nephrectomy, partial nephrectomy, radical cystectomy, dismembered pyeloplasty, and ureteral reconstructive surgery); (b) a codified technique for RAKT [13, 16]; (c) a structured modular training in RAKT, including e-learning, simulation, and dry lab and wet lab training on animal models [32]; (d) the availability of a multidisciplinary team (composed by urologists, anesthesiologists, nephrologists, radiologists, as well as operating room support staff and nurses) with experience in KT and robotic surgery; and (e) the opportunity to perform RAKT at nighttime and/or during the weekend in a dedicated operating room [18].

### 3.3 Selection criteria for RAKT from deceased donors

Following the University of Florence, recipient's exclusion criteria for RAKT from deceased donors include the following: (a) age < 18 years; (b) severe comorbidities with contraindication for robotic surgery; (c) significant atherosclerotic plaques at the level of external iliac vessels; (d) highly complex vascular graft anatomy (likely to require multiple anastomoses); (e) multiple previous abdominal surgeries; and (f) previous KT. A key element of the RAKT program from deceased donor is also represented by the decision-making process aiming to assess the feasibility of RAKT in light of the patient-, graft-, and robotic team-related factors [18] (**Figure 9**). As such, the decision to proceed with an "emergency" RAKT from a deceased donor relies on a careful balance of the potential advantages of robotic surgery (for both the patient and the surgeon) and the logistical challenges of setting up the operating room and the robotic surgical team in a fixed timeframe, respecting the recipient's selection criteria and the maximal thresholds of cold ischemia time. Specifically, planning RAKT from deceased donors follows a pre-specified decision-making process. First, after the alert of a kidney offer is addressed to our transplant team by the Regional Allocation Centre, the surgeon in charge considers the opportunity to perform RAKT according to his/her personal experience and the availability of an expert bedside assistant as well as an expert robotic operating room nursing staff. Then, after the recipient is admitted to the nephrology unit for the pretransplant clinical work-up (which systematically includes a computed tomography angiogram of the abdomen to check for severe atherosclerotic plaques at the external iliac vessels), the surgeon checks that the recipient's inclusion criteria are met. Subsequently, the robotic operating room is checked for availability (even during weekends, at nighttime, and potentially during daytime, if elective non-oncologic robotic procedures can be safely rescheduled), ensuring that the bench surgery starts within 16 hours from the beginning of cold storage of the kidney. Finally, at the time of bench surgery, the graft is carefully inspected to ensure no exclusion criteria for RAKT is present (i.e., highly complex vascular anatomy requiring multiple vascular anastomoses).

### 3.4 The University of Florence technique for RAKT from deceased donors

A step-by-step overview of our surgical technique for RAKT from deceased donors is shown in **Figures 10–12**.

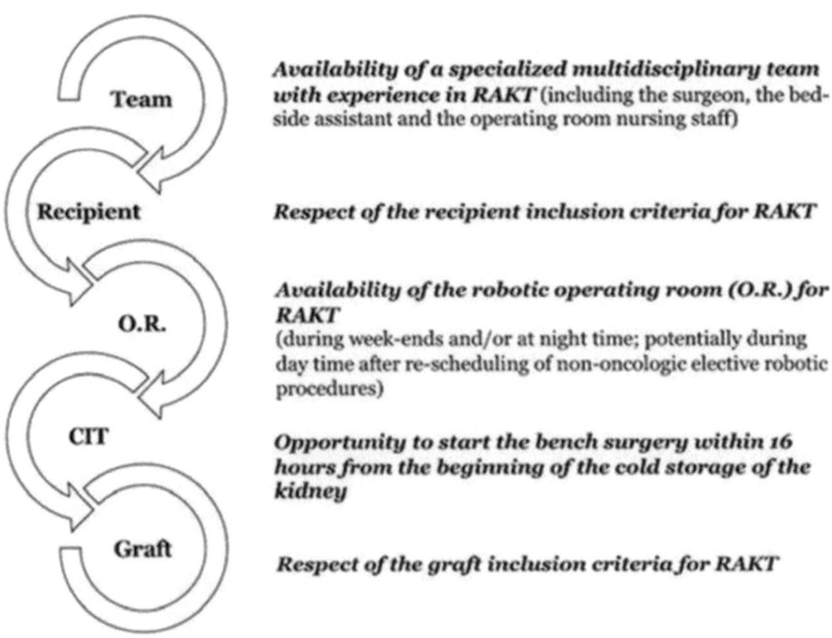


**Figure 9.**
*Flow-chart depicting the decision-making process for RAKT from deceased donors.*

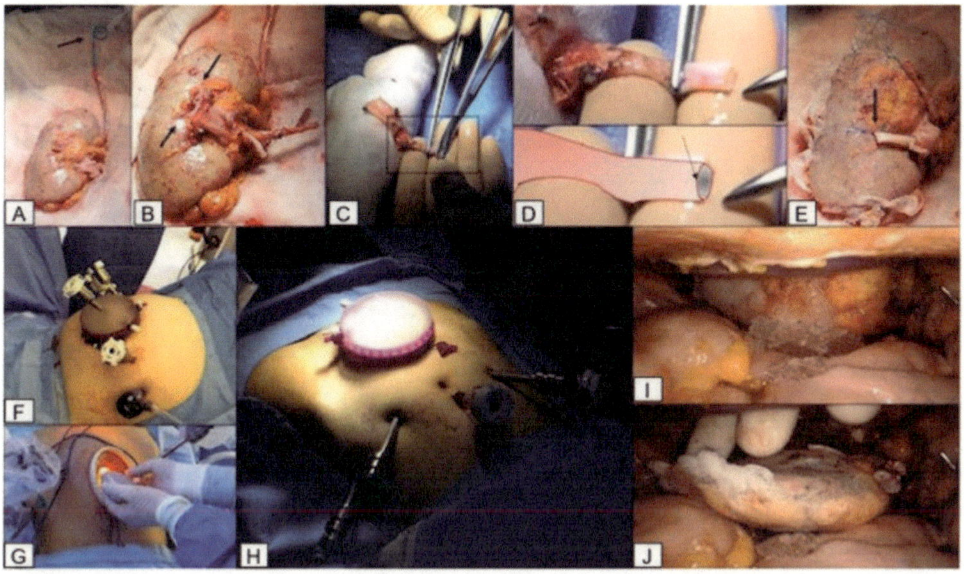


**Figure 10.**
*Overview of the main steps for bench surgery (A-E), port placement (F-H) and insertion of the graft into the abdominal cavity (I, J) during RAKT from deceased donors.*

All procedures were performed with the da Vinci Si® or Xi® robotic platform in a four-arm configuration with a zero-degree lens and one assistant port [18], by a single surgeon (G.V.) with extensive experience in robotic urologic surgery and open KT. The pneumoperitoneum pressure was set at 8 mm using the AirSeal® system, while the Trendelenburg was tilted at 20° in all cases.

The robotic instruments employed for RAKT included the following: (a) large needle driver; (b) black diamond micro-forceps; (c) monopolar curved scissors; (d) Maryland bipolar forceps; (e) prograsp forceps; and (f) robotic bulldog clamps. Laparoscopic instruments included a needle driver, the suction device, laparoscopic scissors, Hem-o-lok (Weck Surgical Instruments, Teleflex Medical, Durham, NC) clips and clip applier, Johan grasping forceps, and the drop-in ultrasound probe.

For insertion of the graft inside the abdominal cavity [13, 16], we employ the GelPOINT® or the Alexis® wound retractor (Applied Medical, Rancho Santa Margarita, CA) through a Pfannenstiel incision (**Figure 10**). Regional hypothermia is achieved by cooling the graft with ice slush introduced through the GelPOINT® via modified Toomey syringes, as previously described [13, 16].

Intraoperative indocyanine green (ICG) fluorescence videography (IFV) (i.e., FireFly® technology) is used to assess the graft and ureteral reperfusion [33, 34].

Abdominal organ procurement is performed according to established principles for donors after brain death (DBD) [35], while specific protocols were followed in the case of donors after circulatory death (DCD) [36]. In this setting, the kidneys are preserved in a hypothermic machine perfusion device (LifePort Kidney Transporter® (Organ Recovery Systems Inc. Chicago, USA)) before transplantation.

During bench surgery (**Figure 10**), the graft is perfused with Celsior® solution and inserted in a gauze jacket filled with ice (and closed with 4–5 stiches) after placement of a 6F, 14 cm double-J stent. Two landmark stiches are placed on the upper and lower sides of the graft vein, while one landmark stich is placed on the upper side of the graft artery, to facilitate the subsequent orientation of the graft inside the abdominal cavity. Finally, the graft artery is modeled to facilitate subsequent intracorporeal arterial anastomosis.

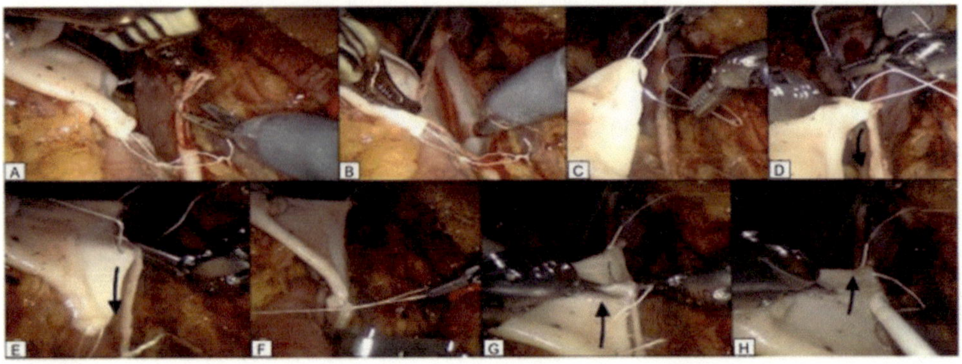


**Figure 11.**
*Overview of the main steps for venous anastomosis during RAKT from deceased donors. (A) A 1–2 cm venotomy is performed on the external iliac vein. (B) The lumen of the external iliac vein is flushed with heparinized saline. (C–F) The graft renal vein is anastomosed in an end-to-side continuous fashion to the external iliac vein using a 6/0 Gore-Tex®. (G and H) The running suture is completed at the caudal angle.*

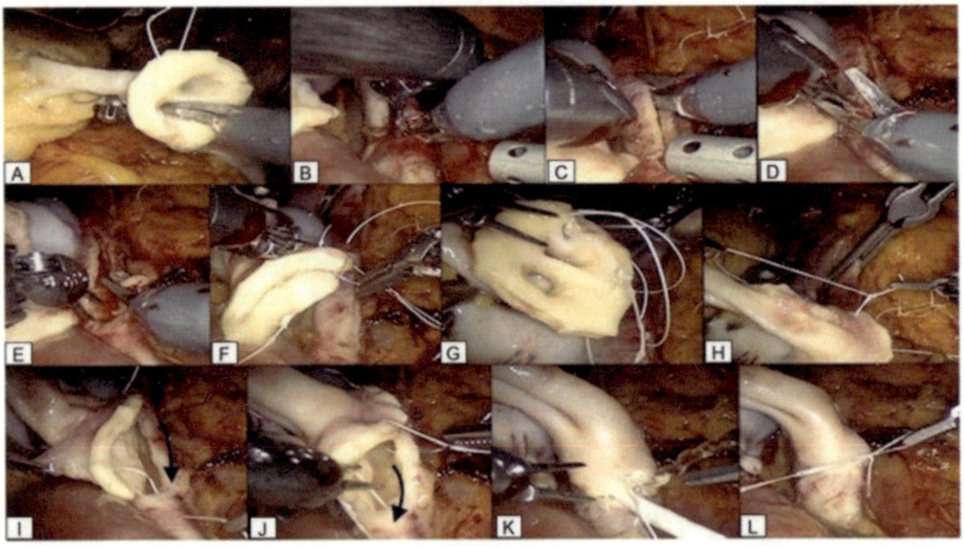


**Figure 12.**
*Overview of the main steps for arterial anastomosis during RAKT from deceased donors. (A-E) A linear arteriotomy is performed and converted into a circular arteriotomy with cold scissors. (F-L) The renal artery is anastomosed in an end-to-side fashion to the external iliac artery using a 5/0 Gore-Tex suture on a CV-6 TTc-9 needle with two running sutures.*

RAKT from deceased donors at our Institution follows the principles of the Vattikuti-Medanta technique [13], adopted by all other centers included in the ERUS-RAKT group [16].

Of note, this technique allows performance of a *transperitoneal* RAKT with final retroperitonealization of the graft after kidney reperfusion.

After induction of general anesthesia, port placement, and docking of the da Vinci Si/Xi robotic platform, the iliac vessels are dissected and prepared for subsequent anastomoses. Then, an extraperitoneal pouch is created, and access is gained into the Retzius space in order to prepare the bladder for subsequent ureteroneocystostomy [18].

Then, a Pfannenstiel incision is performed, and the GelPOINT® device or the Alexis® wound retractor is set in place. The graft is subsequently introduced into the abdominal cavity and the robot is redocked. After achievement of regional hypothermia, a venotomy is performed, the lumen of the external iliac vein is flushed with heparinized saline, and the venous anastomosis is completed in an end-to-side fashion using a 6/0 Gore-Tex suture on a CV-6 TTc-9 needle (**Figure 11**). After additional graft cooling, a liner arteriotomy is performed and converted into a circular arteriotomy with cold scissors. The renal artery is then anastomosed in an end-to-side fashion to the external iliac artery using a 5/0 Gore-Tex suture on a CV-6 TTc-9 needle with two running sutures (**Figure 12**).

After the integrity of the anastomoses is tested, the graft is revascularized and inspected for color and turgor. Intraoperative Doppler ultrasound with the TilePro® feature is employed to check for graft reperfusion in case the da Vinci Si robotic platform is used. On the contrary, if the da Vinci Xi® platform is available, graft and ureteral reperfusions are assessed using intraoperative indocyanine green (ICG) fluorescence videography (IFV) [33]. Then, the graft is allocated in the extraperitoneal pouch, which is partially closed by reapproximating the previously prepared peritoneal flaps with a V-lock running suture or single Hem-o-lok clips. This step avoids graft torsion, facilitates postoperative graft monitoring, and allows convenient access for ultrasound-guided transplant renal biopsy and/or placement of nephrostomy tubes, if needed [37]. Interestingly, we recorded a laminar perirenal fluid collection in almost all patients at ultrasound examinations during the first postoperative period (i.e., postoperative days 1 and 7 and at hospital discharge). However, subsequent follow-up evaluations showed a progressive reduction of this fluid collection until complete reabsorption within 20–30 days after surgery, confirming the complete retroperitonealization of the graft [37].

The last step of the procedure is the ureterovesical anastomosis, which is performed according to a modified Lich-Gregoire technique over the double-J stent. The ureter is anastomosed to the bladder mucosa with two 4.0 Monocryl running sutures; then the detrusor muscle is closed creating an anti-reflux mechanism.

The technique for RAKT from deceased donors evolved over time throughout the learning curve [34]. In particular, few technical nuances have been introduced, according to the surgeon's preference and skills, with the aim to improve the esthetic result and the cost-effectiveness of RAKT, as well as to optimize critical steps such as the assessment of graft and ureteral reperfusion before ureterovesical anastomosis [38].

These technical modifications include insertion of the graft into the abdominal cavity through a Pfannenstiel incision (rather than a periumbilical incision), to improve the esthetic result of RAKT and facilitate the positioning of the graft in the pelvis close to the iliac vessels.

Second, the placement of the GelPOINT® device is achieved *after* preparation of iliac vessels, bladder, and extraperitoneal pouch, to make sure not to injure the bladder while positioning the GelPOINT® device through the Pfannenstiel incision. Of note, in the case of recipients with autosomal dominant polycystic kidney disease (ADPKD), all ports are positioned approximately 3 centimeters downward on the same lines to obtain an increased working space in the right iliac fossa far from the enlarged polycystic kidneys [38].

While mirroring the Vattikuti-Medanta technique, the steps of venous and arterial anastomoses differ slightly from those originally described by the ERUS-RAKT group [18]. In all cases of right-sided grafts, an inferior vena cava (IVC) cuff is used during bench surgery to increase the length of the graft renal vein to facilitate the subsequent venous anastomosis. However, according to our experience in RAKT using right-sided grafts from living donors, the use of an IVC cuff does not appear to be mandatory, as the robotic platform facilitates the performance of a tension-free venous anastomosis even in case of short renal veins.

The venotomy is performed using the standard curved scissors (rather than the *Potts* scissors), and the venous anastomosis is completed in a two-step fashion: first, the posterior plate is closed using a running suture from 12 to 6 o'clock position;

then, a knot is tied, and the anterior plate is completed with a second running suture with the same thread from 6 to 12 o'clock position (**Figure 11**). Tying the knot at 6 o'clock position after completion of the posterior plate may be key to reduce the tension on the anterior plate of the anastomosis, tailoring it according to the graft vein shape and length.

Similarly, the technique for arterial anastomosis follows the principles of the Vattikuti-Medanta technique [13, 16] with key technical nuances in case of deceased donors. First, the arteriotomy is achieved using standard cold scissors (rather than using the aortic punch). Second, due to the increased risk of atherosclerotic plaques and/or calcifications at the level of the external iliac arteries, the arterial anastomosis is performed using two different threads (**Figure 12**). First, the posterior plate of the anastomosis is closed using a running suture from 12 to 6 o'clock position, without tying a knot at 6 o'clock position. Then, the anterior plate is closed in a similar fashion with a running suture from 12 to 6 o'clock position using a second thread. Finally, the two free ends of the threads are tied together at 6 o'clock position, after checking the integrity of the anastomosis. This technique allows to tailor the tension of the anastomosis according to the stiffness and characteristics of both the renal and iliac vessels.

Third, the arterial anastomosis during RAKT from deceased donors is performed using a slightly thicker thread (Gore-Tex 5/0 instead of 6/0).

A specific challenge in case of RAKT from deceased donors is represented by the management of the Carrel's patch for arterial anastomosis. At the beginning of our robotic program for deceased donor RAKT [18], after careful bench surgery showing no significant atherosclerotic plaques at the level of the renal artery ostium, we performed the anastomosis using the Carrel's patch (**Figure 12**). However, with increasing experience the anastomosis is increasingly being performed *without* the Carrel's patch. While in few cases at the beginning of the program, the surgeon had to remove the patch due to the presence of significant atherosclerotic plaques, in the following cases, the Carrel's patch was removed intentionally during bench surgery, and the anastomosis was performed mirroring the technique adopted for living donor RAKT. From a technical point of view, and thanks to the robotic platform, removing the Carrel's patch may provide significant advantages for the surgeon. These include (a) the opportunity to perform a shorter arteriotomy; (b) a more anatomic anastomosis, thanks to the similar caliber of the graft renal artery and external iliac artery; and (c) the reduced risk of atherosclerotic plaques at the level of the graft renal artery (as compared to Carrel's aortic patch).

Finally, a specific technical modification proposed by our group for RAKT from deceased donors is represented by the use of intraoperative indocyanine green (ICG) fluorescence videography (IFV) to assess graft and ureteral reperfusion [33, 34]. The tips and tricks for the use of this technique during RAKT from deceased donors are discussed in the previous publications [18, 33, 34]. In brief, a bolus of 0.3 mg/kg of ICG dissolved in 5% glucose (2 mg/ml) is administered intravenously after completion of vascular anastomoses to allow performance of a real-time qualitative and potentially quantitative assessment of graft and ureteral fluorescence signal [34]. Forty seconds after ICG injection, the camera is switched to reveal fluorescence at the level of vascular anastomoses and the renal parenchyma and ureter to check for their reperfusion, allowing to adapt the ureteral length according to the fluorescence signal to reduce the chance of postoperative ureteral strictures.

### 3.5 RAKT from deceased donors: preliminary results

Overall, 32 RAKTs have been performed at the University of Florence from January 2017 (22.4% of all KT in this period).

The first RAKT from a deceased donor was performed in August 2017. Of the 32 RAKT performed so far, 19 (59.4%) were from deceased donors (n = 5 [26%] from DCD donors; n = 14 [74%] from DBD donors).

Interestingly, thanks to the structured RAKT program developed at the University of Florence, the proportion of RAKT increased over time in the last 3 years, being 18.3%, 26.4%, and 24% of all KT in 2017, 2018, and 2019, respectively. Similarly, the proportion of RAKT from deceased donors increased over time, being 11.1% in 2017, 19.6% in 2018, and 14.3% in 2019 of all KT from deceased donors.

The University of Florence group very recently published their results on their first 17 RAKTs from deceased donors [18]. They now performed 19 cases, all successfully completed without need of open conversion.

The da Vinci Si and Xi robotic platform was used in 15 (79%) and 4 (21%) cases, respectively. In the vast majority of cases (n = 17), RAKT was performed in the right iliac fossa.

The graft was introduced using the GelPOINT® device (or the Alexis® port) in 14 (73.7%) cases through a Pfannenstiel incision, while in 5 (26.3%) through a periumbilical incision.

They recorded one case of intraoperative complication (intraoperative bleeding not requiring transfusion) that required positioning of an additional 5 mm port to increase exposure and help aspiration. Three patients (16%) suffered a high-grade (Clavien-Dindo grade 3) complication (transplant renal artery stenosis requiring percutaneous angioplasty in one patient; percutaneous placement of a nephrostomy tube for hydronephrosis in one patient and transplant renal artery thrombosis requiring graft nephrectomy).

A progressive improvement of renal function was recorded at all time points during the postoperative period. Median eGFR at hospital discharge (median 12 days post-op) was 47.2 ml/min/1.73m$^2$ (IQR 28.9–59.4), while median eGFR at a median follow-up of 15 months was 58.6 ml/min/1.73m$^2$ (IQR 40.0–80.4).

Overall, five (26%) patients required dialysis during the first postoperative week. Of these, one patient due to primary nonfunction after RAKT from an uncontrolled DCD donor; one patient due to graft nephrectomy due to arterial thrombosis; one patient for suspected acute rejection treated with intravenous corticosteroids; and two patients for DGF.

At a median follow-up of 15 months, all patients are alive, and two patients are still on dialysis.

### 3.6 RAKT from deceased donors: future perspectives

We developed the first structured program of RAKT from deceased donors worldwide.

Despite being preliminary, our experience confirms the feasibility of RAKT in this donation setting in centers with a solid background in open KT and robotic surgery and after proper standardized modular training.

From a logistical perspective, RAKT from deceased donors poses specific challenges, which require a comprehensive, multidisciplinary effort to redesign the management strategy of the institution's transplantation pathway. In this view, a highly trained and committed surgical team, as well as the opportunity of a dedicated flexible robotic operating room, are key elements for the success of the program.

The perioperative and functional data in our preliminary series are promising but warrant further investigation. In particular, larger studies with longer follow-up are needed to confirm the safety of RAKT from deceased donors (especially DCD donors), to evaluate the impact of learning curve on patient outcomes, and to identify the predictors of adverse perioperative events (i.e., major surgical complications, PNF and DGF) to refine patient selection.

Yet, extending the number of robotic transplantations performed by centers experienced in robotic surgery using grafts from deceased donors would be key to increase the pool of patients who may benefit from minimally invasive surgery. Notably, this is a critical step toward the definition of evidence-based indications for RAKT in this clinical scenario also from a Guideline's perspective [39].

We entirely share Dr. Alcaraz and colleagues' perspective that "although major improvements in outcomes for transplant patients are likely to come from the field of immunology, small, measurable improvements may yet be possible via technical advances" [40]. As such, we believe RAKT, which is likely to be increasingly performed by referral transplant centers worldwide, may provide unique opportunities for both patients and surgeons, allowing to improve the precision and reduce the morbidity of this procedure. To move the field forward, implementing RAKT programs from deceased donors is the most compelling clinical unmet need for the transplant and urological community.

## 4. Robot-assisted kidney autotransplantation (RAKAT)

### 4.1 History and background

In 1902 Ullmann [41] and Carrel [42] experimentally achieved the first successful animal kidney autotransplantation (KAT), moving the kidney of a dog from its lumbar fossa to its neck, in this way laying the foundations for future kidney (auto) transplantation. In 1956, the Brazilian Campos Freire [43] attempted KAT for the first time on a man with a renal artery aneurysm, although an early thrombosis forced him to perform a nephrectomy. In 1961, Shackman and Dempster repeated this in a case of unilateral renal artery stenosis but with unsatisfactory results [44]. It was not until 1963 when JD Hardy et al. achieved the first successful KAT in human in a case of high ureteral stricture after a large aortic aneurysm repair [45]. McLaughlin et al. demonstrated its utility in the management of complex renal lesions. Following these pioneering surgeries, KAT was adopted as a method to perform renal artery angioplasty in treating hypertension caused by severe renal artery stenoses. In these vascular cases, the ureter was usually not transected; the vascular pedicle is reconstructed in or close to the abdominal incision with subsequent vascular reimplantation on the iliac vessels, making this actually a renal transposition. Only when the indication concerns primary ureteral pathology or when the kidney needs complex surgery on the bench table (and both the vascular pedicle and the ureter are sectioned and subsequently reimplanted), the term KAT is correct. Nowadays, most renovascular problems are treated with endovascular methods, and the indications for KAT have been shifted more toward managing complex ureteral strictures or malignant pathologies for which endoluminal or in vivo repair is impossible or contraindicated. Less frequent indications include loin pain hematuria syndrome, retroperitoneal fibrosis, and metabolic stone disease [46].

KAT is an important surgical last resort technique in order to spare the kidney in select cases. It allows ex vivo management of complex renal or ureteral pathology, which would not be treatable with conventional techniques, without resulting in important kidney function loss. For this purpose, the harvested kidney is cooled on ice slush and flushed with an ice-cold preservation solution during bench surgery, thus reducing tissue oxygen requirement.

Traditionally, KAT has been performed through a large midline laparotomy, a large paramedian extraperitoneal incision or the combination of a lumbotomy for the nephrectomy phase with a lower abdominal incision for the transplantation phase; thus being a very invasive procedure, and, albeit having a low mortality rate (1.3%), postoperative morbidity may be as high as 46.2%. Due to the historic invasiveness of the procedure, and the unfamiliarity of many urologists with the field of KT, KAT has never gained much popularity and often these kidneys were sacrificed. However, since the introduction of laparoscopy in urology, attempts have been made to reduce the morbidity of open KAT. Fabrizio et al. [47] described in 2000 the first laparoscopic nephrectomy for KAT; however, the patient still required a periumbilical incision for extraction of the graft and a pelvic incision for the transplantation [47]. Today, the most accepted approach is to perform laparoscopic nephrectomy, via a three-port transperitoneal access, and open KAT, using the classical Gibson incision for both extraction and introduction of the graft, resulting in possible low complication rate and excellent long-term autograft function [48].

In recent years, due to the success of RAKT, interest is rising to reevaluate KAT as an ultimate nephron-sparing option in complex cases. In 2014, Gordon et al. published the first case of robot-assisted kidney autotransplantation (RAKAT) to treat extensive ureteral loss after complicated ureterorenoscopy for ureterolithiasis [49]. They used a completely intracorporeal technique, establishing in vivo hypothermic renal perfusion by continuous renal artery irrigation. The robot was redocked between nephrectomy and transplantation phase, and the table was repositioned rather than the patient. The complete intracorporeal technique was successfully repeated by Lee et al. [50] in 2015. Despite these promising results, the totally intracorporeal technique is not suitable in patients where ex vivo bench repair is required (e.g., multiple vessel grafts, complex oncological cases, lithiasis treatment) or where the surgeon would prefer to transplant the autograft in the contralateral iliac fossa (e.g., disturbed pelvic vascular anatomy or excessive fibrosis). In the same period, Sood et al. theoretically described a technique for RAKAT using extracorporeal tabletop graft reconstruction, using a GelPOINT device, in order to broaden indications of RAKAT [51]. In 2017, Araki et al. [52] published a case using this extracorporeal RAKAT technique in a patient with proximal ureteral stenosis. Also in 2017, Decaestecker et al. [53] performed the first extracorporeal RAKAT in Europe and to date have the largest series of RAKAT worldwide. This European series also adopted a totally intracorporeal technique.

### 4.2 Operative technique

Decaestecker et al. published the largest series of RAKAT worldwide, all for non-oncological cases [53]. Their technique is based on the experience within the ERUS-RAKT working group, as described by Breda et al. [16], and on the theoretical report by Sood et al. [51]. We will describe the extracorporeal bench work technique and the totally intracorporeal technique with the da Vinci Si® and Xi® robotic platform.

#### *4.2.1 Extracorporeal bench work technique (video)*

##### *4.2.1.1 Trocar and patient position*

**Figures 13** and **14** describe the patient and trocar positioning for Si and Xi, right or left, during nephrectomy and transplantation phase.

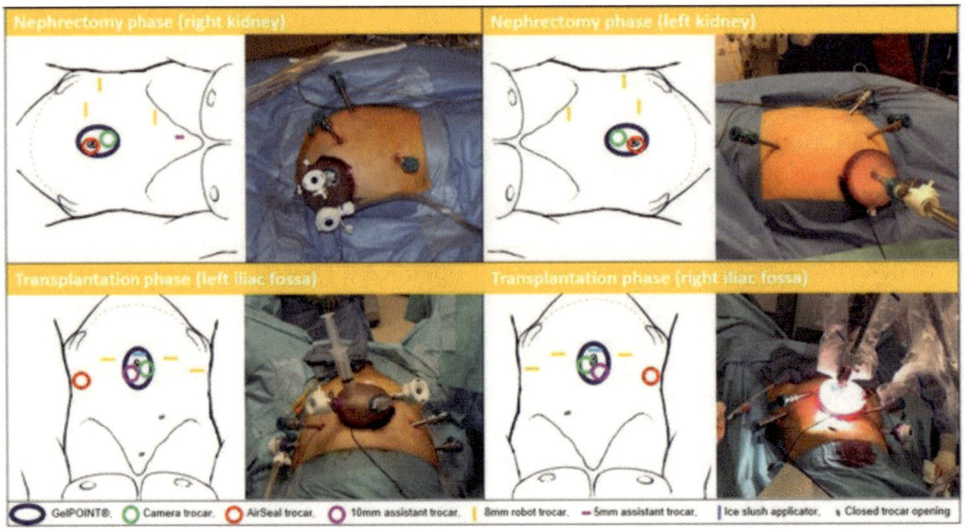


**Figure 13.**
*Trocar and patient positioning for extracorporeal RAKAT using Si. Nephrectomy phase: patient in lateral decubitus; GelPOINT® through a 6 cm vertical peri-umbilical incision containing camera and assistant trocar; three 8 mm robot trocars in hemiabdomen, one subcostal and 2 in the iliac fossa. Transplantation phase: patient repositioned in lithotomy position, legs in Allen stirrups, table in 20–30° Trendelenburg; three 8 mm robotic trocars in the lower abdomen, reusing the 2 former iliac fossa trocar sites. Low-pressure pneumoperitoneum realized with the AirSeal®System.*

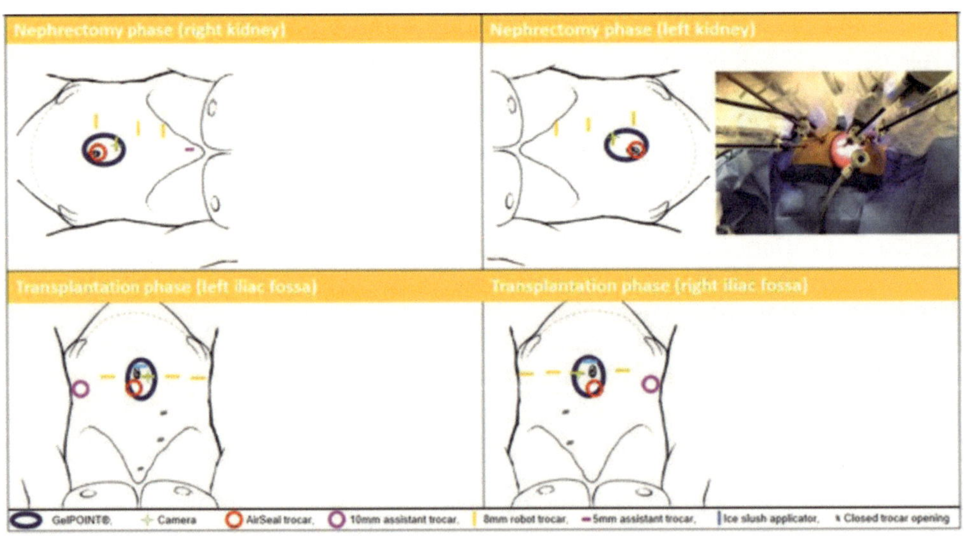


**Figure 14.**
*Trocar and patient positioning for extracorporeal RAKAT using Xi. Nephrectomy phase: patient in lateral decubitus; GelPOINT® through a 6 cm vertical peri-umbilical incision containing robot and assistant trocar; three 8 mm robot trocars in hemiabdomen on a slightly oblique line, 2 subcostal and 1 in the iliac fossa. Transplantation phase: patient repositioned in lithotomy position, table in 20–30° Trendelenburg; three 8 mm robotic trocars in the lower abdomen, reusing 1 former iliac fossa trocar site. Low-pressure pneumoperitoneum realised with the AirSeal®System.*

#### *4.2.1.2 "Donor" nephrectomy*

A "donor" nephrectomy is performed with the patient in the lateral decubitus position, maximizing the renal vessel length and transecting the ureter just proximal of the strictured segment or at the level of the crossing with the iliac vessels. After administering 2500–5000 units of heparin intravenously according to the weight of the patient, the renal vessels are transected after securing the vessels with either a laparoscopic/robotic vascular stapler or double clipping the vessels with Click'aV plus® clips (Grena, Amsterdam, the Netherlands, Europe), followed by a transfixing ligation of the clipped vascular stump with Prolene® 5/0 (Ethicon Inc., Johnson & Johnson Corp, Cincinnati, OH, USA) to prevent clip slipping. The latter is done robotically after the kidney is exteriorized by the table-side assistant through the GelPOINT®.

#### *4.2.1.3 Bench work*

Upon retrieval, the graft is immediately perfused on the bench with 4° Celsius preservation solution (Institut Georges Lopez-1®). If necessary, bench vascular reconstruction can be performed for duplicated renal arteries (end-to-side reconstruction of the lower pole to main artery or pantaloon reconstruction of two central arteries). During cold storage, tabletop flexible ureterorenoscopy or nephroscopy can be performed to extract nephro- or ureterolithiasis. The kidney is wrapped in an ice gauze jacket with a central hole exposing the renal hilum (**Figure 15**).

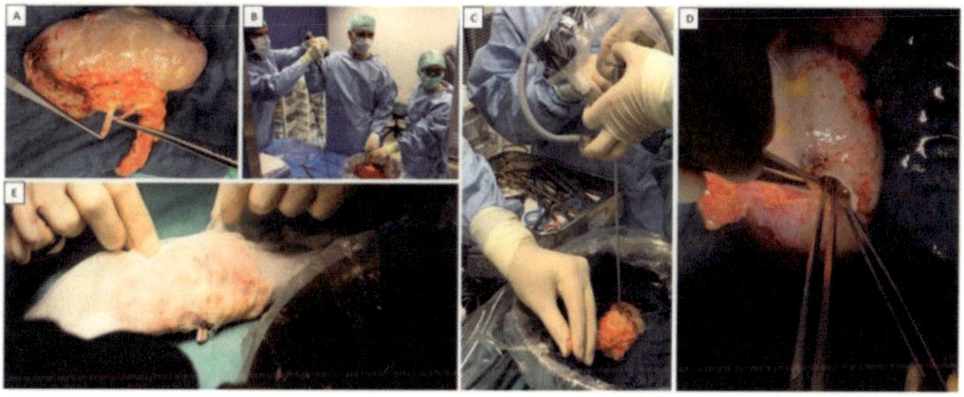


**Figure 15.**
*Bench work in extracorporeal RAKAT technique. (A) End-to-side anastomosis of lower pole artery on main renal artery. (B) Extraction of nephrolithiasis. (C) Nephroscopy. (D) Extraction of lithiasis from calyceal diverticulum and closing diverticulum infundibulum. (E) Wrapping of the kidney in ice gauze jacket, leaving opening for the structures.*

#### *4.2.1.4 Transplantation phase*

During cold storage, the robot is undocked, the incisions are temporarily closed, and the patient is repositioned in lithotomy position (Si/X) or dorsal decubitus (Xi). For the transplantation phase, the robot is redocked, and RAKT is performed following the Vattikuti-Medanta technique as previously described and adopted by the ERUS-RAKT group. With the extracorporeal technique, the kidney is usually transplanted to the contralateral iliac fossa unless the proximal ureter of the graft is absent or very short and urges a ureteropyelostomy (native distal ureter to transplant pyelum) or uretero-ureterostomy (native distal ureter to transplant ureter). The iliac vessels can be very hard to dissect due to excessive fibrosis caused by previous surgery and/or radiotherapy.

*4.2.2 Totally intracorporeal technique*

*4.2.2.1 Selection of patients*

The totally intracorporeal technique is not suitable in patients where ex vivo bench repair is required (e.g., multiple vessel grafts, complex oncological cases, lithiasis treatment) and might be less optimal in cases where the surgeon would prefer to transplant the autograft in the contralateral iliac fossa (e.g., disturbed pelvic vascular anatomy or excessive fibrosis).

*4.2.2.2 Trocar and patient position*

**Figures 16** and **17** describe the patient and trocar positioning for Si and Xi, right or left, during nephrectomy and transplantation phase. Note that the GelPOINT® device is not used and as much trocars as possible are reused, although some need to be exchanged for each other. For the transplantation phase, the patient is positioned on the PinkPad® (Kebomed, Apeldoorn, the Netherlands, Europe) in a modified lateral flank position using inflatable pressure bags. Together with maximal side tilting of the table (15°), the patient is in a 65° flank position which makes nephrectomy feasible. After nephrectomy and intracorporeal flushing, the robot needs to be undocked, and the table is repositioned rather than the patient (from maximal side tilt to contralateral maximal side tilt, partially) deflating the pressure bags to bring the patient more or less horizontal and adding 20–30° of Trendelenburg). Using the Si/X system, the robot needs to

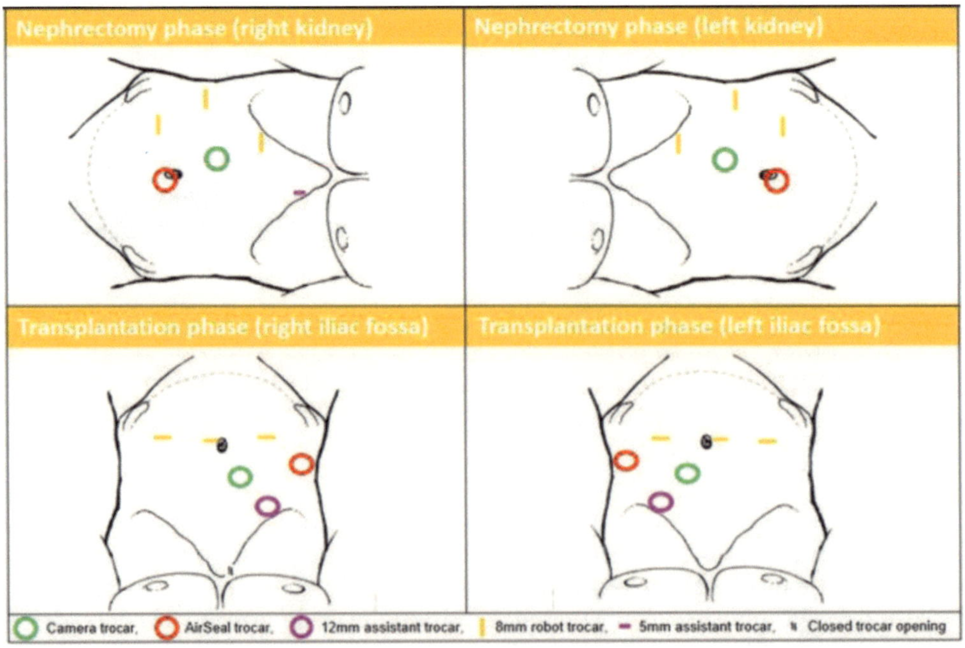


**Figure 16.**
*Trocar and patient positioning for RAKAT intracorporeal technique Si. No use of GelPOINT® device. Nephrectomy phase: patient positioned in lateral decubitus; camera trocar supra-umbilical, three 8 mm robot trocars in hemiabdomen, AirSeal trocar as assistant trocar infra-umbilical. Transplantation phase: robot undocked, table repositioned rather than the patient, and robot redocked (side-docking next to left leg); three 8 mm robotic trocars in the lower abdomen, reusing 1 former caudal robot trocar site and AirSeal trocar site; AirSeal in flank position reusing former robot trocar site; assistant trocar subcostal reusing former robot trocar site.*

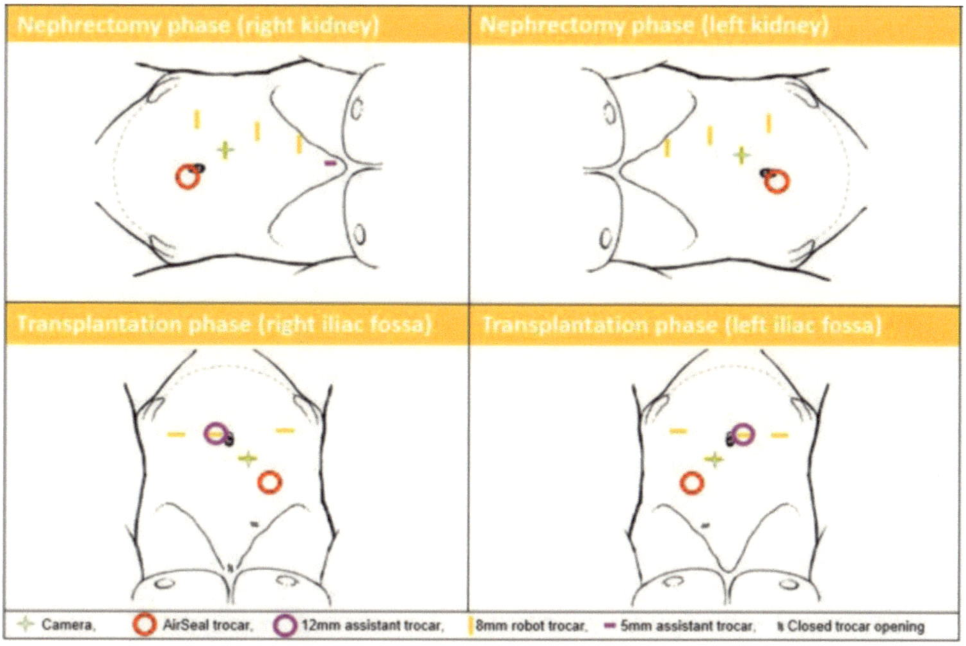


**Figure 17.**
*Trocar and patient positioning for RAKAT intracorporeal technique Xi. No use of GelPOINT® device. Nephrectomy phase: patient positioned in lateral decubitus; camera trocar supra-umbilical, three 8 mm robot trocars in hemiabdomen, AirSeal trocar as assistant trocar infra-umbilical. Transplantation phase: robot undocked, table repositioned rather than the patient, and robot redocked (side-docking next to left leg); three 8 mm robotic trocars in the lower abdomen, reusing 1 former caudal robot trocar site and AirSeal trocar site; AirSeal in flank position reusing former robot trocar site; assistant trocar subcostal reusing former robot trocar site.*

be repositioned from flank-docking tot side-docking; using the Xi system, only the boom needs to be rotated 90° before redocking. In case of expected pelvic fibrosis, it is wise to prepare the iliac vessels before clamping the renal hilum in order to reduce intracorporeal "cold" ischemia time as well as the amount of intracorporeal cold fluid that could potentially lower central body temperature. This means that three phases with two repositions are necessary. The Xi system with easy docking and repositioning of the boom and integrated table motion is a real advantage for these challenging cases.

#### *4.2.2.3 "Donor" nephrectomy*

During nephrectomy, more fat is left on the lower pole of the kidney in order to be able to manipulate the kidney intracorporeally. Care should also be taken to skeletonize the renal vessels and gain adequate length as would normally be performed on the bench. After clamping the renal vessels, they are not transected, but incised to introduce a 5–7 Fr Fogarty catheter with open tip to flush the kidney intracorporeal with 4°C physiologic NaCL solution until the effluent is clear. Note that any solution containing potassium should not be used in order to prevent hyperkalemia and possible arrhythmias by peritoneal reabsorption. After flushing, the renal vessels are transected, and the Fogarty is blocked in the renal artery lumen with inflating the balloon with 0.5–1 cc. The kidney is now continuously flushed at a low flow rate with the intention of intravascular cooling but preventing lowering body temperature by excessive flushing. Effective flushing can be confirmed continuously by looking for renal vein effluent. The kidney is repositioned from flank to pelvis, and the robot is redocked for table repositioning.

#### *4.2.2.4 Transplantation phase*

The venous anastomosis is performed in the same way as for the extracorporeal technique. Flushing (and graft cooling) through the renal artery is continued until the venous anastomosis is complete. The Fogarty is removed, and the arterial anastomosis is performed, resulting in only 10—15 min of rewarming time. With the intracorporeal technique, the kidney is usually transplanted to the ipsilateral iliac fossa.

### *4.2.3 Results*

Decaestecker et al. published their initial experience on 7 patients [53], updated their results of the first 10 cases at EAU 2019 congress [54], and now performed 15 cases, making this the largest reported series worldwide. Thirteen cases were performed extracorporeally and two intracorporeally. Ureteral stricture disease was the main indication (12/15). All 15 RAKATs were successfully completed without intraoperative complications needing open conversion. Compared to pre-op, there was a significant decrease in mean serum creatinine ($p = 0.027$) and a nonsignificant increase of mean overall and autotransplant GFR estimated by nuclear DMSA and Cr-EDTA scans at 3 months post-op. All patients were free from indwelling catheters or nephrostomy tube, recurrent urinary tract infections, debilitating stent symptoms, flank pain, or macroscopic hematuria at the last follow-up. Short hospital stay and early recovery confirmed the minimal invasiveness of the approach although 3/15 patients experienced a high-grade complication (pulmonary embolism, wound dehiscence, and lower limb compartment syndrome without lasting disability). Of note is that the high-grade complications occurred in former cancer patients that had the combination of multiple surgeries and radiotherapy.

## 5. Learning curve and training

The learning curve for RAKT can be relatively short for surgeons experienced in robotic surgery and kidney transplant surgery [25, 26]. It cannot be stressed enough that a high level of robotic experience is recommended before starting this kind of high-stake surgery. Training the technique on dry and wet lab models is mandatory. The structured RAKT course provided at ORSI Academy [32] is recommended as well as an experienced RAKT proctor supporting first cases. In this way a safe introduction of this new technique is possible.

## 6. Conclusions

RAKT has been proven to be an advanced application for KT. The technique is now standardized, and surgical data show that RAKT is safe, feasible, and reproducible when performed by surgeons with experience in both robotic and KT surgery. Most experience has been gained with grafts from living donors, but RAKT from deceased donors is feasible taking into account careful selection and optimizing logistics. Finally, RAKAT is an extension of the RAKT technique and is a minimal invasive way to salvage kidneys with complex renal, vascular, or ureteral pathology, which cannot be treated with conventional in situ techniques. Although the ultimate goal could be intracorporeal RAKAT, the extracorporeal technique is more versatile for complex cases. Training and proctoring are key to safely introduce this advanced robotic technique and give the transplant patient population the advantages of a minimal invasive approach for KT.

## Acknowledgements

This chapter has been written on behalf of the European Association of Urology Robotic Urology Section (ERUS) robot-assisted kidney transplantation (RAKT) working group chaired by Alberto Breda. We want to thank all the members and associates of the ERUS-RAKT working group: Antonio Alcaraz, Paolo Fornara, Alberto Breda, Sergio Serni, Volkan Tugcu, Karel Decaestecker, Giampaolo Siena, Nicolas Doumerc, Michael Stöckle, Alessandro Volpe, Graziano Vignolini, Ravi Barod, Angelo Territo, Riccardo Campi, Mireia Musquera, Liesbeth Desender, and Francesc Vigués.

## Conflict of interest

The authors declare no conflict of interest.

## Author details

Karel Decaestecker[1*], Angelo Territo[2], Riccardo Campi[3,4], Benjamin Van Parys[1], Giulio Bevilacqua[2], Liesbeth Desender[1] and Alberto Breda[2]

1 Ghent University Hospital, Ghent, Belgium

2 Fundaciò Puigvert, Autonoma University of Barcelona, Spain

3 Department of Urological Robotic Surgery and Renal Transplantation, Careggi Hospital, University of Florence, Florence, Italy

4 Department of Experimental and Clinical Medicine, University of Florence, Florence, Italy

*Address all correspondence to: karel.decaestecker@uzgent.be

## References

[1] Collins AJ, Foley RN, Gilbertson DT, Chen SC. United States renal data system public health surveillance of chronic kidney disease and end-stage renal disease. Kidney International. Supplement. 2015;**5**(1):2-7. DOI: 10.1038/kisup.2015.2

[2] Herrell SD, Smith JA. Laparoscopic and robotic radical prostatectomy: What are the real advantages? BJU International. 2005;**95**(1):3-4. DOI: 10.1111/j.1464-410X.2005.05235.x

[3] Territo A, Mottrie A, Abaza R, Rogers C, Menon M, Bhandari M, et al. Robotic kidney transplantation: Current status and future perspectives. Minerva Urologica e Nefrologica. 2017;**69**(1):5-13. DOI: 10.23736/S0393-2249.16.02856-3

[4] Ratner LE, Ciseck LJ, Moore RG, et al. Laparoscopic live donor nephrectomy. Transplantation. 1995;**60**:1047-1049

[5] Horgan S, Vanuno D, Benedetti E. Early experience with robotically assisted laparoscopic donor nephrectomy. Surgical Laparoscopy, Endoscopy & Percutaneous Techniques. 2002;**12**(1):64-70. DOI: 10.1097/00019509-200202000-00011

[6] Hubert J, Renoult E, Mourey E, Frimat L, Cormier L, Kessler M. Complete robotic-assistance during laparoscopic living donor nephrectomies: An evaluation of 38 procedures at a single site. International Journal of Urology. 2007;**14**(11):986-989. DOI: 10.1111/j.1442-2042.2007.01876.x

[7] Renoult E, Hubert J, Ladrière M, Billaut N, Mourey E, Feuillu B, et al. Robot-assisted laparoscopic and open live-donor nephrectomy: A comparison of donor morbidity and early renal allograft outcomes. Nephrology, Dialysis, Transplantation. 2006;**21**(2):472-477. DOI: 10.1093/ndt/gfi150

[8] Cohen B, Smits JM, Haase B, Persijn G, Vanrenterghem Y, Frei U. Expanding the donor pool to increase renal transplantation. Nephrology, Dialysis, Transplantation. 2005;**20**(1):34-41. DOI: 10.1093/ndt/gfh506

[9] Banasik M. Living donor transplantation--the real gift of life. Procurement and the ethical assessment. Annals of Transplantation. 2006;**11**(1):4-6

[10] Bettschart V, Boubaker A, Martinet O, Golshayan D, Wauters JP, Mosimann F. Laparoscopic right nephrectomy for live kidney donation: Functional results. Transplant International. 2003;**16**(6):419-424. DOI: 10.1007/s00147-003-0561-y

[11] Kumar A, Chaturvedi S, Gulia A, Maheshwari R, Dassi V, Desai P. Laparoscopic live donor nephrectomy: Comparison of outcomes right versus left. Transplantation Proceedings. 2018;**50**(8):2327-2332. DOI: 10.1016/j.transproceed.2018.03.034

[12] Giulianotti P, Gorodner V, Sbrana F, Tzvetanov I, Jeon H, Bianco F, et al. Robotic transabdominal kidney transplantation in a morbidly obese patient. American Journal of Transplantation. 2010;**10**(6):1478-1482. DOI: 10.1111/j.1600-6143.2010.03116.x

[13] Menon M, Sood A, Bhandari M, Kher V, Ghosh P, Abaza R, et al. Robotic kidney transplantation with regional hypothermia: A step-by-step description of the vattikuti urology institute-medanta technique (IDEAL phase 2a). European Urology. 2014;**65**(5):991-1000. DOI: 10.1016/j.eururo.2013.12.006

[14] Breda A, Gausa L, Territo A, et al. Robotic-assisted kidney transplantation: Our first case. World Journal of Urology. 2016;**34**(3):443-447

[15] Doumerc N, Roumiguié M, Rischmann P, Sallusto F. Totally robotic approach with Transvaginal insertion for kidney transplantation. European Urology. 2015;**68**(6):1103-1104. DOI: 10.1016/j.eururo.2015.07.026

[16] Breda A, Territo A, Gausa L, Tuğcu V, Alcaraz A, Musquera M, et al. Robot-assisted kidney transplantation: The European experience [figure presented]. European Urology. 2018;**73**(2):273-281. DOI: 10.1016/j.eururo.2017.08.028

[17] Territo A, Gausa L, Alcaraz A, Musquera M, Doumerc N, Decaestecker K, et al. European experience of robot-assisted kidney transplantation: Minimum of 1-year follow-up. BJU International. 2018;**122**(2):255-262. DOI: 10.1111/bju.14247

[18] Vignolini G, Campi R, Sessa F, Greco I, Larti A, Giancane S, et al. Development of a robot-assisted kidney transplantation programme from deceased donors in a referral academic Centre: Technical nuances and preliminary results. BJU International. 2019;**123**(3):474-484. DOI: 10.1111/bju.14588

[19] Siena G, Campi R, Decaestecker K, Tuğcu V, Sahin S, Alcaraz A, et al. Robot-assisted kidney transplantation with regional hypothermia using grafts with multiple vessels after extracorporeal vascular reconstruction: Results from the European Association of Urology robotic urology section working group. European Urology Focus. 2018;**4**(2):175-184. DOI: 10.1016/j.euf.2018.07.022

[20] Spinoit AF, Moreels N, Raes A, Prytula A, De Groote R, Ploumidis A, et al. Single-setting robot-assisted kidney transplantation consecutive to single-port laparoscopic nephrectomy in a child and robot-assisted living-related donor nephrectomy: Initial Ghent experience. Journal of Pediatric Urology. 2019;**15**:578-579. DOI: 10.1016/j.jpurol.2019.08.005

[21] Giacomoni A, Di Sandro S, Lauterio A, Concone G, Buscemi V, Rossetti O, et al. Robotic nephrectomy for living donation: Surgical technique and literature systematic review. American Journal of Surgery. 2016;**211**(6):1135-1142. DOI: 10.1016/j.amjsurg.2015.08.019

[22] Shahbazov R, Maluf D, Azari F, Hakim D, Martin O, Dicocco P, et al. Laparoscopic versus finger-assisted open donor nephrectomy technique: A possible safe alternative. Experimental and Clinical Transplantation. 2019. DOI: 10.6002/ect.2019.0115

[23] Dols LFC, Kok NFM, Ijzermans JNM. Live donor nephrectomy: A review of evidence for surgical techniques. Transplant International. 2010;**23**(2):121-130. DOI: 10.1111/j.1432-2277.2009.01027.x

[24] Levi Sandri GB, de Werra E, Mascianà G, Guerra F, Spoletini G, Lai Q. The use of robotic surgery in abdominal organ transplantation: A literature review. Clinical Transplantation. 2017;**31**(1). DOI: 10.1111/ctr.12856

[25] Rampersad C, Patel P, Koulack J, McGregor T. Back-to-back comparison of mini-open vs. laparoscopic technique for living kidney donation. Canadian Urological Association Journal. 2016;**10**(7-8 August):253-257. DOI: 10.5489/cuaj.3725

[26] Menon M, Abaza R, Sood A, Ahlawat R, Ghani KR, Jeong W, et al. Robotic kidney transplantation with regional hypothermia: Evolution of a

novel procedure utilizing the IDEAL guidelines (IDEAL phase 0 and 1). European Urology. 2014;**65**(5):1001-1009. DOI: 10.1016/j.eururo.2013.11.011

[27] Bianchi G, Martorana E, Ghaith A, Pirola GM, Rani M, Bove P, et al. Laparoscopic access overview: Is there a safest entry method? Actas Urológicas Españolas (English Ed). 2016;**40**(6):386-392. DOI: 10.1016/j.acuroe.2016.05.011

[28] Breda A, Territo A, Gausa L, Rodríguez-Faba O, Caffaratti J, de León JP, et al. Robotic kidney transplantation: One year after the beginning. World Journal of Urology. 2017;**35**(10):1507-1515. DOI: 10.1007/s00345-017-2006-8

[29] Wagenaar S, Nederhoed JH, Hoksbergen AWJ, Bonjer HJ, Wisselink W, van Ramshorst GH. Minimally invasive, laparoscopic, and robotic-assisted techniques versus open techniques for kidney transplant recipients: A systematic review. European Urology. 2017;**72**(2):205-217. DOI: 10.1016/j.eururo.2017.02.020

[30] Ahlawat RK, Tugcu V, Arora S, Wong P, Sood A, Jeong W, et al. Learning curves and timing of surgical trials: Robotic kidney transplantation with regional hypothermia. Journal of Endourology. 2018;**32**(12):1160-1165. DOI: 10.1089/end.2017.0697

[31] Sood A, Ghani KR, Ahlawat R, Modi P, Abaza R, Jeong W, et al. Application of the statistical process control method for prospective patient safety monitoring during the learning phase: Robotic kidney transplantation with regional hypothermia (ideal phase 2a-b). European Urology. 2014;**66**(2):371-378. DOI: 10.1016/j.eururo.2014.02.055

[32] Breda A, Decaestecker K, Territo A. Robotic Kidney Transplantation Course, Orsi Academy, Belgium. Available from: https://www.orsi-online.com/en/training/rkt-w-dr-breda

[33] Vignolini G, Sessa F, Greco I, Cito G, Vanacore D, Cocci A, et al. Intraoperative assessment of ureteral and graft reperfusion during robotic kidney transplantation with indocyanine green fluorescence videography. Minerva Urologica e Nefrologica. 2019;**71**(1):79-84. DOI: 10.23736/S0393-2249.18.03278-2

[34] Cacciamani GE, Shakir A, Tafuri A, Gill K, Han J, Ahmadi N, et al. Best practices in near-infrared fluorescence imaging with indocyanine green (NIRF/ICG)-guided robotic urologic surgery: A systematic review-based expert consensus. World Journal of Urology. 2019. DOI: 10.1007/s00345-019-02870-z

[35] Figueiredo A, Lledò- Garcìa E. European Texbook on Kidney Tranplantation (ESTU-EAU). The European Association of Urology First ed. Arnhem: The EAU section of transplantation urology; 2017

[36] Peris A, Lazzeri C, Cianchi G, Bonizzoli M, Batacchi S, Franci A, et al. Implementing a donation after circulatory death program in a setting of donation after brain death activity. Minerva Anestesiologica. 2018;**84**(12):1387-1392. DOI: 10.23736/S0375-9393.18.12635-6

[37] Campi R, Vignolini G, Savi E, Sessa F, Agostini S, Serni S. Robotic kidney transplantation allows safe access for transplant renal biopsy and percutaneous procedures. Transplant International. 2019. DOI: 10.1111/tri.13517

[38] Vignolini G, Sessa F, Greco I, Pili A, Giancane S, Sebastianelli A, et al. Robotic kidney transplantation from a brain-dead deceased donor in a patient with autosomal dominant polycystic

kidney disease: First case report. Journal of Endourology Case Reports. 2018;**4**(1):124-128. DOI: 10.1089/cren.2018.0050

[39] Kälble T, Alcaraz A, Budde K, Humke U, Karam G, Lucan M, et al. European Association of Urology : Guidelines on renal transplantation. European Urology. 2005;**47**:156-166

[40] Alcaraz A, Peri L, Izquierdo L, Musquera MI. Robotic kidney transplant the near future? European Urology. 2017;**72**(2):218-219. DOI: 10.1016/j.eururo.2017.03.018

[41] Ullman E. Experimentelle Nierentransplantation. 1902. Wiener Klinische Wochenschrift. 2002;**114**(4):126-127

[42] Carrel D. La Technique Opératoire Des Anastomoses Vasculaires Et La Transplantation Des Viscères. Lyon Médical. 1964;**212**:1561-1568

[43] Campos Freire G. Personal communication to J. J. Kaufman. Transactions of the American Association of Genito-Urinary Surgeons. 1966;**58**:108

[44] Schackman R, Dempster WY. Surgical kidney. A case demonstrated at the PostGraduate medical School of London. British Medical Journal. 1924

[45] Hardy JD. High ureteral injuries: Management by autotransplantation of the kidney. JAMA. 1963;**184**(2):97-101. DOI: 10.1001/jama.1963.03700150051008

[46] Azhar B, Patel S, Chadha P, Hakim N. Indications for renal autotransplant: An overview. Experimental and Clinical Transplantation. 2015;**13**(2):109-114. DOI: 10.6002/ect.2014.0238

[47] Fabrizio MD, Kavoussi LR, Jackman S, Chan DY, Tseng E, Ratner LE. Laparoscopic nephrectomy for autotransplantation. Urology. 2000;**55**(1):145. DOI: 10.1016/S0090-4295(99)00367-2

[48] Tran G, Ramaswamy K, Chi T, Meng M, Freise C, Stoller ML. Laparoscopic nephrectomy with autotransplantation: Safety, efficacy and long-term durability. The Journal of Urology. 2015;**194**(3):738-743. DOI: 10.1016/j.juro.2015.03.089

[49] Gordon ZN, Angell J, Abaza R. Completely intracorporeal robotic renal autotransplantation. The Journal of Urology. 2014;**192**(5):1516-1522. DOI: 10.1016/j.juro.2014.02.2589

[50] Lee JY, Alzahrani T, Ordon M. Intra-corporeal robotic renal auto-transplantation. J Can Urol Assoc. 2015;**9**(9-10 October):E748-E749. DOI: 10.5489/cuaj.3015

[51] Sood A, Ghosh P, Jeong W, Khanna S, Das J, Bhandari M, et al. Minimally invasive kidney transplantation: Perioperative considerations and key 6-month outcomes. Transplantation. 2015;**99**(2):316-323. DOI: 10.1097/TP.0000000000000590

[52] Araki M, Wada K, Mitsui Y, Sadahira T, Kubota R, Nishimura S, et al. Robotic renal autotransplantation: First case outside of North America. Acta Medica Okayama. 2017;**71**(4):351-355. DOI: 10.18926/AMO/55313

[53] Decaestecker K, Van Parys B, Van Besien J, Doumerc N, Desender L, Randon C, et al. Robot-assisted kidney autotransplantation: A minimally invasive way to salvage kidneys. European Urology Focus. 2018;**4**(2):198-205. DOI: 10.1016/j.euf.2018.07.019

[54] Van Parys B, Van Besien J, Doumerc N, Desender L, Randon C, De Ryck F, et al. Mp76-15 robot-assisted kidney autotransplantation (Rakat): Update from the first series in Europe. The Journal of Urology. 2019;**201**(Suppl 4). DOI: 10.1097/01.ju.0000557307.93315.cc